"Now...tell me how the 'three-date rule' works."

She'd read about it herself. Quite possibly in a magazine.

"It does what it says on the tin," she said. "You get three dates and that's it. Both parties know the rules in advance so it keeps things casual and makes it easy to back off but stay friends, if that's what either party wants."

"Sounds perfect," Lachlan said thoughtfully. "So...what about the subclauses?"

"Like what?"

"What constitutes a 'date'? And...is sex on the agenda? On the first date, even, given that the time limit's going to be rather restricted? I mean, this is kind of like 'friends with benefits' but with a use-by date, yes?"

Oh... Pippa couldn't respond to the query. He'd said the *s* word, and her brain had turned to absolute mush. She was staring at Lachlan's hands, for heaven's sake. Imagining what it would be like to have his fingers trailing over her skin. It felt like it could be dangerous. They might leave a flicker of tiny flames in their wake...

Dear Reader,

I have to confess that I adore London. I lived there for eighteen months when I was a child. My dad worked at Hammersmith Hospital and we lived near Primrose Hill, close enough to the zoo to hear the animals at night. I've visited London many times since then and I fell in love with Richmond long ago, on my visits to see my editors when the Mills & Boon/Harlequin offices were—appropriately, I thought—on Paradise Road.

Anyway...I love a chance to set a story in London. I've created a hospital in Richmond, and the gorgeous park is an important part of my hero's background—a background that's dark enough to make him quite sure nobody can steal his heart. Lachlan hasn't factored in meeting Pippa, however. And she has no idea that Lachlan is about to change her life. She has every intention of protecting herself and even comes up with rules that cannot be broken.

Even if they both want to.

Maybe *especially* if they both want to.

Happy reading!

With love,

Alison xxx

MIDWIFE'S
THREE-DATE RULE

ALISON ROBERTS

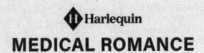

MEDICAL ROMANCE

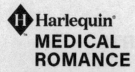

Harlequin®
MEDICAL ROMANCE

ISBN-13: 978-1-335-94298-2

Midwife's Three-Date Rule

Copyright © 2025 by Alison Roberts

Harlequin Enterprises ULC
22 Adelaide St. West, 41st Floor
Toronto, Ontario M5H 4E3, Canada
www.Harlequin.com

Printed in U.S.A.

Alison Roberts has been lucky enough to live in the South of France for several years recently but is now back in her home country of New Zealand. She is also lucky enough to write for the Harlequin Medical Romance line. A primary school teacher in a former life, she later became a qualified paramedic. She loves to travel and dance, drink champagne, and spend time with her daughter and her friends. Alison Roberts is the author of over one hundred books!

Books by Alison Roberts

Harlequin Medical Romance

A Tale of Two Midwives

Falling for Her Forbidden Flatmate
Miracle Twins to Heal Them

Daredevil Doctors

Forbidden Nights with the Paramedic
Rebel Doctor's Baby Surprise

Morgan Family Medics

Secret Son to Change His Life
How to Rescue the Heart Doctor

Paramedics and Pups

The Italian, His Pup and Me

Therapy Pup to Heal the Surgeon
City Vet, Country Temptation
Paramedic's Reunion in Paradise

Visit the Author Profile page
at Harlequin.com for more titles.

CHAPTER ONE

'WHO *IS* THAT?'

Philippa Gordon could feel her gaze being drawn and then caught, despite the fact that her attention had been centred on the staff huddle gathering in front of the whiteboard at the back of the central nurses' station for the shift hand-over. The ward receptionist was talking to new arrivals at the desk—an anxious-looking, heavily pregnant woman in a wheelchair and her even more anxious-looking partner. Other incoming night shift midwives and support staff were busy chatting and finding notepads and pens.

Pippa didn't realise she'd spoken aloud until Sally, who was updating boxes on the whiteboard, glanced over her shoulder.

'New consultant,' she said. 'Lachlan Smythe. Starts tomorrow.'

'What's he doing here at this time of day, then? It's seven p.m.'

'Moving into his office, I believe.'

A second glance was irresistible—and it

wasn't simply because this man was more than attractive enough to invite second glances. *This* was the famous Lachlan Smythe who, according to the hospital grapevine, had been headhunted from a top job in a major American hospital for the sought-after HoD position at The Queen Mary Hospital's Birthing Centre.

Pippa had a legitimate reason to be watching him now. She would be working with the man, after all.

'Younger looking than I expected,' she murmured.

'*Better* looking than *I* expected,' Sally whispered back. 'Lucky us. I met him earlier. He seems very nice.' She looked past Pippa. 'Everybody ready? I'd like to get started so that some of us can head home on time for once.'

There was a chorus of assent and a shuffle as some people took chairs and others crowded closer.

'Right… Room One, we have Mary McGovan. She's forty-one weeks gestation; G4 P3 so she knows what she's doing. No red flags. Came in at eighteen hundred hours and currently six centimetres dilated. Suzie, you've got a student midwife with you tonight, so this should be a perfect introduction.'

Pippa took one more glance as the new HoD passed the reception desk. Mr Smythe's CV was apparently notable for the number of prestigious hospitals he'd worked in, his cutting-edge research projects and an impressive list of peer-reviewed articles in leading medical journals. No wonder he had such a confident air about him— as though he already felt as if he belonged here.

She hoped he was as 'nice' as Sally believed. Their last HoD had, unfortunately, been one of those old school surgeons who was inclined to dismiss the opinions of staff members who were further down the pecking order, like nurses or midwives. She could feel the corners of her mouth curling upwards a little. It had to be a good sign that he was carrying that large cardboard box himself instead of finding a porter to shift his belongings. Especially when it looked like an awkward and rather heavy burden. It had to be an effort so it was a surprise to see him suddenly turning his head over the top of the box.

Oh, Lord...

Pippa knew the feeling that someone was watching you and how it could send a shiver down your spine. When it was strong enough to make you turn it was usually because it felt creepy enough to make the hairs on the back of your neck stand up, and here she was with a smile on her face, probably *looking* creepy. Hastily, she straightened her face and turned to focus on Sally and the whiteboard. She wasn't quite fast enough, however. For just a heartbeat there, they'd made eye contact that *she* could feel, even at this distance.

What was *that* about?

Pippa took note of the rooms assigned to her that included an older woman, Linda, having her first baby at the age of forty-two after IVF intervention, and Helen, who had been admitted at three centimetres dilated, with regular contractions, but was slow to progress. As one of the most experienced midwives on the shift, she was being assigned to any labour that could be potentially more complicated. She'd already lost any interest in the new boss she had yet to meet. These women were the reason she was here and each one of them would remind her of why she was so passionate about this job.

'Room Six, Stella Braithwaite. Thirty-six years old, twenty-one weeks gestation, G2, P+1. Came in at sixteen hundred hours and is having intermittent contractions. Ultrasound and monitoring suggest they're Braxton Hicks and the cervix is closed but she's understandably very anxious so we're keeping her in and doing thirty-minute obs. Pippa, I've put her on your list, too.'

Okay…maybe some women and their stories were more of a reminder than others. The '+1' designation meant that Stella had lost her first baby before the twenty-four-week mark and that put her at much higher risk of losing a second baby. It wasn't just Pippa's professional interest that was captured by this case.

This was personal.

Stella was the first person on her list that she went to introduce herself to as the handover finished. Her heart went out to the woman who was lying stiffly on the bed as if she was too afraid to move a muscle. As Pippa knocked and entered the room quietly, both Stella and her partner were staring at the screen of the CTG monitor beside the bed and Pippa knew that they were watching the lines forming and listening to every blip of their baby's heartbeat.

She'd been there. Too many times. She knew that fear.

'I'm Pippa,' she introduced herself. 'I'll be looking after you tonight, Stella.'

Stella nodded.

Her partner was holding her hand tightly. 'I'm Tony,' he said.

Pippa took in the information on the screen of the monitor. 'That's looking very reassuring,' she said.

'Is it?' Stella sounded doubtful. 'Are you sure?'

'I'm sure.' Pippa picked up the thin strip of graph paper that was pooling on the floor to run between her hands and see what had been recorded recently. 'Did someone explain what we're keeping an eye on?'

'The baby's heart rate,' Stella said. 'If it slows down or gets irregular, it's a concerning sign.'

'And that bottom line is the strength of the contractions,' Tony added. 'If they get stronger it means it's likely to be real labour starting and not those false contractions.'

'Braxton Hicks.' Pippa nodded. She was still rapidly scanning the graph paper. 'We measure contractions in millimetres of mercury—like a blood pressure. If it's real labour, they'll be between forty and sixty millimetres. The strongest one I can see here is no more than fifteen millimetres. And they're getting further apart.' She smiled at Stella—aiming for a mix of reassurance and encouragement. 'I know it's not easy, but try and relax. Stress—and fatigue—are both triggers for Braxton Hicks.'

She couldn't miss the look that Stella and Tony exchanged.

'What is it?' she asked.

Stella bit her lip.

'She thinks this is her fault,' Tony admitted.

'What?' Pippa was horrified. 'Of course it isn't.'

'That's what I keep telling her.'

'But Pippa said that stress can trigger it.' Stella's eyes filled with tears that spilled over. 'I tried not to get stressed. I really did but…but…'

It was Tony who filled the silence. 'We're at exactly the same day it was when we lost our first baby,' he said. His voice cracked. 'Twenty-one weeks and three days.'

Oh…

Pippa had to pull in a deep breath. To find that courage that she knew she had, despite—or perhaps because of—knowing exactly what that would have been like. It was termed a late miscarriage because the baby was too early to survive. It was referred to as a foetus and it would have fitted into the palms of their hands but it would have *looked* like a real baby. And it would have hurt beyond measure.

She sank onto the edge of the bed and reached for Stella's other hand. 'I totally understand how stressful this is,' she said. 'But there's absolutely no sign that it's about to happen again. The CTG is normal. Your ultrasound was normal. You're very close to being past the day you were dreading and we're going to be here to look after you until you feel more confident. Now…have you both had something to eat since you came in?'

They both shook their heads.

'I can recommend our cafeteria, which will be open for another couple of hours. They do a really good lasagne. Or you could get sandwiches and have a picnic. I'll be coming in to see you whenever I can but you can push your buzzer any time and, if I can, I'll come straight away.' She gave Stella's hand a squeeze and stood up. 'I'd better go and do some work now.'

The next person on her list was only two rooms away and she begged for an update on her dilation status as soon as Pippa introduced herself.

Within minutes, she was the second woman to burst into tears in front of Pippa.

'You've got to be kidding. I'm only *halfway*?' Her head flopped back onto the pillows. The hand holding the mouthpiece of the Entonox cylinder hit the mattress. 'I thought I could this,' she moaned. 'But now I don't think I can. Terry's fed up, too. He went to find some food ages ago and he hasn't even bothered coming back yet.'

'Six centimetres is good,' Pippa said. 'It's past halfway and it's progress. You were only three when you came in.'

'That was *hours* ago.'

There were tears streaming down Helen's face now. 'But I'd been having contractions for fifteen hours before I even came in. *Fifteen* hours! I'm so tired. And it hurts...'

'I know.'

'Do you?' Helen glared at her. 'How many kids have you got?'

'I haven't got any of my own.'

Oh, boy…this was clearly going to be one of those nights with too many poignant reminders of the past. She'd had plenty of practice keeping it hidden, however, and still managed to find a smile for Helen.

'I've lost count of how many babies I've helped into the world, though,' she added with a smile. 'So, I do know a lot about it.'

'It'll be worse when it's your turn,' Helen said. 'You'll see.'

Pippa stripped off her gloves and stood up from where she'd been perched on the side of the bed to do the internal examination. She was only in her mid-thirties so why wouldn't people make the assumption that she was just putting off motherhood? What would it be like in ten years' time when people might start thinking she was selfish because she'd never wanted to have kids, or worse—feeling sorry for her because she couldn't?

'You really are doing well, Helen,' she said. 'And baby's still coping with the contractions, but I'd like to leave the monitor on for a bit longer unless you want to get up.'

Helen's head shake was miserable and Pippa took hold of her hand. The slow progress of this labour was clearly beginning to take a significant emotional toll and that was something that had to be taken into consideration in the management of this baby's arrival. 'Maybe I should get one of our doctors to come and have a chat to you about what we could do to help?'

'Like what?'

'More pain relief might let you get a bit of rest. Some sleep, even. You might want to have another think about having stronger medication or an epidural. Or an infusion to help make the contractions stronger.'

'But I said I don't want drugs. Or an epidural. I wanted to have a natural birth.'

'I know.' Pippa was sympathetic. 'Maybe you'd like to try the pool again? Or the birth ball? Or walking around?'

Helen shook her head again. 'I'm too tired.'

'When did you last have a wee?' Pippa asked.

'I can't remember.'

'It's really important,' Pippa said. 'If your bladder's full it can make it harder for baby's head to descend and it can slow things down by making the contractions less effective and more painful.' She reached for the chart on the end of the bed to see if the midwife who'd been with Helen on the day shift had recorded the information.

'*Oww…*' Helen's loud groan, as a new contraction started, seemed like agreement with what Pippa was telling her. She pulled the mouthpiece close enough to suck in a deep breath of the mix of nitrous oxide and oxygen.

Helen spat out the mouthpiece as the contraction ended.

'I *have* changed my mind,' she groaned. 'I just want this baby out. *Please*...'

'I'll find someone to come and see you,' Pippa said.

She found Sandy, the consultant on duty tonight, at the nurses' station, hanging up on an internal phone call.

'We're down one anaesthetist,' she sighed. 'There's some horrible gastric bug going around and she's had to go home. The staff shortage might mean we can only have one theatre open tonight and we've already got a potential C-section waiting in the emergency department and keeping my registrar busy. Fingers crossed we don't get any more. Could be a long night.'

'At least we've got a new consultant on board from tomorrow.'

'A new Head of Department, even.' Sandy's raised eyebrows made her look hopeful. 'Maybe he'll look at improving our staffing issues.'

For some odd reason, Pippa found herself glancing away from the reception desk. In the direction she'd seen Lachlan Smythe going, carrying that box, a couple of hours ago.

It was highly unlikely he was still in the building.

Even less likely that he'd look at her again and give her that strange impression that he already knew who she was. Or that *she* was the person he'd been waiting to meet?

She shook off the ridiculous notion.

'Have you got a couple of minutes?' she asked Sandy. 'We've got a woman in Room Three. Primigravida, cephalic presentation, but slow progress of just on two centimetres in over four hours. Mother's getting tired and distressed enough to be ready to discuss modifying her birth plan.'

Helen chose to have IV pain relief and her response to the oxytocin infusion that Sandy had offered was rapid. Less than two hours later, she gave birth to a large baby boy who started crying loudly the moment Pippa lifted him up to put on his mother's chest.

'Sounds hungry already,' she said.

'Just like his father, then…' Helen reached to touch her baby but she was smiling up at Terry.

'He's beautiful,' Terry said, swiping tears off his face. 'Just like his mum.'

Pippa clamped the cord and showed Terry how to cut it. She did an Apgar score on the baby and recorded his weight and time of birth.

'He's looking very healthy,' she told the proud parents. 'Have you got a name for him yet?'

'Jack,' Terry said. 'After my dad.'

'One of my favourite names,' Pippa said.

'He's still crying,' Helen said, as she took the baby back into her arms. 'Can I try feeding him?'

'I was just about to suggest that. Look at the way he's turning his head...he's already trying to latch on himself. Put your hand behind his head and bring it up to your nipple and then wait until his mouth is really wide open—like a frog—and put in as much of the nipple as you can. Here... I'll help...'

Baby Jack was sucking within seconds, both parents mesmerised by his talent. It left Pippa free to monitor the third stage of labour, delivering the placenta and checking that it was intact. She had fifteen-minute observations to do on both mother and baby for the first hour after birth and, in that time, Pippa also stitched up the episiotomy that had prevented any serious tearing from the birth of a baby who weighed just over ten pounds.

'There you go, all done.' She smiled at the perfect picture of a brand-new family in front of her, the mother lying back in the circle of the father's arms, the baby asleep in *her* arms. 'I'll leave you in peace for a little while to get to know each other but I'll come back and check on you soon. Ring your bell if you need something before then.'

'Could I get this needle out of my hand before you go?' Helen asked. 'I don't need that infusion now, do I?'

'I'd like it to stay in a bit longer,' Pippa told her. 'But I'll unhook it from the tubing so it won't be such a nuisance.'

Lachlan Smythe leaned back in his chair and checked his watch.

Good grief…it was nearly midnight. It wasn't simply the time it had taken to fill the bookshelf with his textbooks and hang his framed degrees on the walls of his new office—there had been a glitch with getting access to the computer systems he needed and he didn't want to be waiting for someone from the IT department first thing tomorrow morning.

He wanted to hit the ground running. He'd learned, thanks to moving around so much, that it was the best way to get to know a new hospital and his new colleagues. It could make the first few days feel like navigating a professional minefield, for sure, but there was nothing like a good challenge to make you feel really alive, was there?

Lachlan loved his work as an obstetrician.

He'd spent too many years letting his research work and teaching cut into the time he spent doing what he'd put so much passion into learning to do extremely well—helping people realise their dreams of creating their own families and keeping mothers and babies safe during the birthing process. Accepting this position at The Queen Mary Hospital was a step back to the work he loved the most and he couldn't wait to get started, but there was an unexpected tension to this particular appointment.

There was more to this than a purely professional change in his life. He'd grown up here. Not just in London but *here*, in the heart of Richmond.

He glanced at the small photograph in a silver frame that had become a permanent desk ornament after so many years. An image of two adults and two small boys. His family. He'd been eight years old. His brother Liam had been five. They were grinning at each other, while their proud parents beamed at the camera above their heads. Lachlan loved this photo. Because this represented the happiest part of his life. Before any of them knew the horrors of what lay ahead for them all as a family.

Was the importance of this picture partly why he'd chosen to take this new position? Because the memories he knew he could only find in this tiny patch of the planet were the only links he had left to his family?

Maybe…

But professional considerations would, as always, take precedence over anything so personal and it was far too late to be here. If he didn't get a decent sleep he wouldn't be in top form for his first day on the job.

Lachlan left his office and walked towards the doors at the other end of the ward that led out to the elevators and stairwell. Unencumbered with boxes this time, he slowed as he passed the central hub of the ward with its reception desk, banks of computer screens, filing cabinets and the ubiquitous whiteboard.

The whiteboard that he'd seen that staff member standing in front of the last time he'd walked past. He had no idea who she was but she'd been wearing scrubs and a lanyard and was taking part in a shift handover so she had to be one of his new colleagues, but in that moment he'd turned his head she'd been looking directly at *him*.

Smiling at him.

As if she approved of what she was seeing?

It should have been somewhat disturbing but Lachlan decided that it had made him curious. Was she just a smiley sort of person? Maybe he'd get the chance to find out. He'd certainly recognise her easily again. Who wouldn't with that long braid of distinctively red hair?

There was a phone ringing on the desk. Lachlan slowed his pace as he realised there was no one here to answer it.

The area was deserted.

A quick scan of the whiteboard told him that there was an emergency Caesarean underway in Theatre One and that the rest of the staff were probably all occupied in the rooms of a very full ward. He saw the capital letters of the word BORN written across boxes in several different rooms, the most recent of which had been in Room Three.

The phone stopped and immediately began ringing again. He was about to answer it himself when he noticed a digital display beside the whiteboard light up, along with the sound of an alarm.

Room Three, it relayed. Code Red.

Code Red was an urgent call for medical assistance for a patient whose condition was rapidly deteriorating but wasn't yet in a cardiac or respiratory arrest, in which case a crash call would have been made. He wasn't familiar with the response to an alarm like this in The Queen Mary. Would available staff have been bleeped in other areas of the hospital? He couldn't see anyone emerging from rooms to get somewhere else in a hurry.

He was moving himself, however.

Where the hell was Room Three?

She'd been out of the room for less than fifteen minutes. Just long enough to do another set of reassuringly normal observations on Stella and point out that she hadn't had a contraction strong enough to show on the CTG in the last ninety minutes, have a quick bathroom break and scribble an update on the whiteboard to record the birth of a baby in Room Three.

Terry was holding his son as Pippa went back into their room. Helen was lying back on her pillows and she was looking…

…extremely unwell. She was very pale and was that a sheen of perspiration on her face?

'I'm so cold,' she said as soon as Pippa reached her bedside. 'And kind of dizzy. I think I'm going to be sick…'

Pippa grabbed a container and gave it to her. She put her fingers on Helen's wrist to find a pulse that was far too rapid. Her breathing was also rapid and yes…her skin was cool and clammy.

Pippa's own heart rate was increasing noticeably as she flicked back the bedcovers to see a bloodstain that was already large enough to be visible on either side of Helen's body and legs. The absorbent sheet beneath her hips was heavy enough to confirm a sudden, severe blood loss.

'Oh, my God,' Terry whispered. 'What's happening?'

A massive post-partum haemorrhage was what was happening but there was no time to try and explain in any detail right now.

'Helen's losing a bit of blood.'

A lot of blood. Quite possibly a life-threatening amount of blood.

Pippa reached to push the alarm button at the head of the bed to summon emergency assistance.

'I'm going to lie you flat, Helen, and put a mask on to give you some oxygen. And then I'm going to take your blood pressure.'

'I'm scared,' Helen whispered.

'I know, sweetheart.' Pippa was careful to keep her tone calm and reassuring as she moved swiftly. She put a plastic mask over Helen's mouth and nose and turned on the wall supply of oxygen. She reattached the tubing to the IV line and rolled the small wheel to start fluids running again. Then she wrapped a blood pressure cuff around Helen's upper arm. 'Don't worry, we're going to get this sorted,' she said as she pushed a button to start an automatic blood pressure recording.

Pippa was thinking as fast as she was moving. She might have to push the cardiac arrest button to summon the kind of assistance she needed because she'd seen that both the consultant and registrar on duty in the ward tonight were in Theatre with an emergency C-section for a breech presentation baby that had decided to make an appearance earlier than expected.

'I'm going to start massaging your tummy again,' she warned Helen. 'It might be a bit uncomfortable but it looks like your uterus needs a bit more help to shrink properly.'

Helen cried out in pain as Pippa pressed down on the top of the uterus, which was still on the high side for someone who had just given birth. Terry made a distressed sound at the same time. He was pressed against the wall, almost as pale as Helen, clutching the bundle that was baby Jack, who let out his own whimper. The fresh absorbent sheet she had tucked under Helen's hips was already soaked with fresh blood.

Please, Pippa begged silently. *I need help...*

Even as the plea formed in her head, the door was opening...

She would have been happy to see anyone, but she was astonished to see the last person she could have imagined responding to this emergency call.

Lachlan Smythe?

CHAPTER TWO

LACHLAN BARELY REGISTERED that it was the staff member he'd been thinking about only minutes ago as he introduced himself to her—and the frightened-looking man holding a baby. His focus then shifted to the woman on the bed who looked as though her level of consciousness was dropping.

'What's happening?' he asked succinctly, as he rolled up the sleeves of his shirt, thrust his arms into a gown and pulled some gloves from the box on the wall.

The midwife—Pippa, according to her name badge—kept massaging the woman's uterus as she responded.

'PPH. Estimated blood loss at least six hundred mils. Last blood pressure was ninety-six over forty-eight. Heart rate one twenty-six. Pulse ox ninety-seven. Uterus was a bit slow to start contracting but there wasn't any sign of excessive bleeding in the first hour after birth.'

'Background?'

'Primigravida. Labour of more than twenty hours before she accepted any intervention. Large baby born just over an hour ago.'

Lachlan nodded at the information. A long labour and a large baby were both risk factors for a uterus that was simply unable to contract efficiently which was, by far, the most common cause for a post-partem haemorrhage. Trauma and retained tissue also had to be considered.

'Any tears?'

'No. She had an episiotomy that was straight-forward to repair.'

'Was the placenta intact?'

'Yes. It's still here, if you want to check.'

He would, but not now. He moved to the wall phone and punched in a number. He needed to alert the blood bank that they might need to acti-vate a massive transfusion protocol. In the mean-time, he'd need units of whole blood, red blood cells and fresh, frozen plasma. He needed to get an operating theatre on standby in case they couldn't stop the bleeding with drug therapy and massage. He also needed more hands on deck. Pippa was clearly competent and managing an emergency situation impressively calmly but there was a lot that was about to happen. A phys-ical examination of the patient. Drugs needed to be drawn up and administered. Blood samples taken. Constant monitoring of vital signs.

'When did the bleeding start?'

'Within the last twenty minutes. Sudden onset with pallor, diaphoresis and syncope.'

'Is that IV-line patent?'

'I think so.'

'Good. We'll need to get a type and cross-match, stat. IV trolley?'

'Just there.' Pippa nodded towards the wall where the man was now holding a crying baby.

As Lachlan moved the trolley closer to the bed, he took a moment to reassure the man that they were doing what was needed to deal with this complication. As soon as more staff members arrived, he would designate someone to stay with him.

Right now, he had only the midwife Pippa to work with and he had to hope she was as good at her job as she appeared to be on first impressions.

She was taking another set of vital signs. 'Blood pressure's dropped to ninety over forty-five,' she told him quietly. 'And GCS is down to thirteen.'

A dropping level of consciousness took this to a new level of concern. Shock due to blood loss was the leading cause of maternal fatalities.

'We need another IV access,' he said, as he took a blood sample for a type and cross match and full blood count. 'This one's marginal.'

More staff arrived. Lachlan asked the midwife to take a set of vital signs every five minutes and to weigh the soaked absorbent sheets to get a more accurate estimate of blood loss. A support worker was dispatched to get the blood samples to the laboratory as quickly as possible and bring back the units of blood products and he asked Pippa to insert a Foley catheter to ensure that bladder distention wasn't contributing to the failure of the uterus to contract.

Lachlan tried, and failed, to get a cannula into a vein on Helen's hand. Worryingly, the IV line in her other hand looked as if it wasn't patent any longer.

Pippa saw that he was trying to find another palpable vein and handed him an alcohol wipe and then a cannula.

'Can't feel anything,' he said quietly. 'She's as flat as a pancake. I'll give it one more try, but then we'll look at an alternative.'

'A cut down?'

Lachlan shook his head. He was carefully changing direction and depth with the needle but there was no flashback to indicate he was anywhere near a blood vessel.

'Intra-osseus?' Pippa was opening a drawer on the IV trolley.

'No. I'll do an external jugular cannulation. More effective and we can use a larger gauge needle.' Lachlan gave up on the arm. 'Can someone give us a head down tilt for the bed, please, and, Pippa, let's take Helen's pillow away and could you turn her head to the side for me and help her keep as still as possible?'

Pippa was no stranger to high-intensity medical emergency situations although, fortunately, they didn't happen very often and very rarely with as dramatic a presentation as this massive blood loss.

There were more people arriving in the room now. She'd noticed when Terry and baby Jack had been ushered out to be cared for elsewhere and she'd seen the supplies of blood arriving. The on-duty consultant, Sandy, had come down from Theatre, having left her registrar to finish the final suturing after the C-section she had performed but she didn't take over Pippa's assistance for Lachlan. She stood to one side and double-checked that the placenta was intact and there was no retained tissue that could be causing the bleeding.

'You were right, Pippa,' she confirmed. 'I can't see anything missing.'

This wasn't the time but Pippa was aware that she would remember later that it felt good to have her skills recognised, even in a small way, in front of not only a new senior colleague but their incoming HoD. The only thing that mattered right now was doing everything they could to deal with the emergency and Pippa was completely focused on what she was being asked to do. She didn't want her part in this resuscitation to be found wanting in any way.

Sandy could have stepped in at that point and taken over Pippa's position but perhaps she wanted the opportunity to watch the way Lachlan Smythe was managing a life-or-death scenario.

It was quite likely, Pippa thought, that Sandy was just as impressed with his performance as she was herself.

He was so calm.

So in control.

And his clinical skills were faultless. He'd made the cannulation of the large neck vein, which wasn't exactly an everyday procedure, look very easy—even with Helen's low blood volume.

'Pop your finger on the vein for me, would you, Pippa?' The almost casual request had been the only indication that the task was challenging. 'Just above the clavicle. If you occlude it, I'll get a much better target.'

They had been working closely together with the cannulation of the external jugular vein and then the drawing up, checking and administration of more drugs. They were working fast and were close enough for their arms and hands to touch at times, but not because they were getting in each other's way. It felt seamless in fact, as if they'd worked together on many occasions over a long period and yet it had only been minutes since this emergency had unfolded.

It made Pippa remember, for just a heartbeat, that strange frisson when he'd first made eye contact with her. That notion that he'd recognised her. That maybe he knew more about her than she was comfortable with.

Lachlan just seemed quite comfortable as he gave Helen a thorough physical examination to look for any hidden trauma that could be causing the bleeding. He nodded with satisfaction as he palpated her abdomen.

'Uterus is definitely firmer,' he said. 'We're going in the right direction.'

He looked up a short time later to catch Pippa's gaze as she was hanging another unit of blood onto the IV pole.

'Great suturing on that episiotomy,' he said. 'Very neatly done.'

The tension began to fade and Pippa focused on Helen, providing more reassurance as her blood pressure slowly came up enough for her to become more aware of what was happening around her.

'You're doing well,' she assured her, slipping a pillow beneath her head again. 'The bleeding's slowed right down and your blood pressure's coming up. You'll start feeling better very soon.'

'Where's my baby? Where's Jack?'

'Jack's been taken to the nursery so that he can be checked by a paediatrician and looked after until you feel better. Terry's with him. It's okay, Helen. It's all going to be fine.'

And it was. One by one, the extra staff in the room went back to other duties. The standby for Theatre was cancelled and the blood bank informed that the haemorrhage was under control and no further supplies were needed. The intensive care unit was contacted to arrange for Helen to be transferred to receive the intensive monitoring she would need for the next few hours until she could be admitted to a post-natal ward.

'I'll go with her,' Lachlan said. He stripped off his gloves and blood-spattered gown. 'I'd rather do the handover myself.'

Pippa found herself, for the second time tonight, watching this new staff member walk away. It was the middle of the night. Lachlan Smythe wasn't due to officially start work here yet until the morning. He could be going home to his own bed at this point but it felt as if that hadn't even occurred to him.

Yeah…his commitment to his work was definitely impressive.

Pippa was making a mental list of the immediate tasks she had ahead of her as she refocused on her own work. Room Three needed a thorough clean-up and Stella was overdue for her next set of observations. It was quite likely that there would be more deliveries that Pippa could assist with for the rest of this shift, but with a bit of luck she might soon be able to take the proper break she should have had a couple of hours ago.

Talk about jumping in at the deep end.

Lachlan had expected to meet his new colleagues in the controlled environment of a staff huddle and a quiet tour of all the wards that were part of his department. He needed to get familiar with the locations of the operating theatre suite and the outpatient department before his first lists started on his second day on the job and he was hoping for a bit of quiet time to get up to speed with any protocols that might well have been updated since he'd last worked in a UK hospital.

He'd found his way back to the labour ward easily enough after handing over Helen's care to the ICU staff and finding her husband, Terry, to tell him what had happened and reassure him that the emergency was over.

His head was spinning somewhat, in a combination of fatigue and the sense of displacement of being not only in a different work environment but in a different country than he had been only a matter of hours ago. The stress of unexpectedly being in control of a situation that could have ended very differently had been a curve ball, not to mention the number of new people he'd met, spoken to on the phone or worked with. He might have difficulty in remembering every name but he wasn't going to forget how impressed he'd been with the systems in place and such an efficient response from everybody involved, given the time of night and low staffing thresholds.

He certainly wasn't going to forget the person he'd worked most closely with, who'd been the first to start dealing with what was an alarming adverse event that could make even the most experienced medics feel more than a beat of panic.

That midwife.

Pippa.

He didn't know her last name yet, but he fully intended to compliment her on her skills and thank her for her assistance before he went home to try and snatch a few hours' sleep. She'd been brilliant to work with.

Outstanding, in fact.

She'd been doing all the right things before

he'd arrived and then she'd simply slotted in to work with him as if she was totally in sync with the way he worked. As if she was familiar with the way he thought, even. She was calm under pressure and clearly experienced. If he had to guess—although he usually avoided guessing ages when it came to women—he'd put her in her mid-thirties. Was she one of those heroic women who were busy raising their children but still holding down what could be a challenging career? Did she have a supportive husband, perhaps? And a beloved family dog who would be overjoyed to see her arriving home after a long night shift?

Just why he was so curious was too difficult to fathom, probably due to the fuzzy edges that fatigue was giving his thoughts. Maybe that was why he was standing, staring blankly at the whiteboard in the central area of the labour ward. Pippa's name was beside the line for Room Six and the last update had put its occupant into the transitional stage so she was probably busy ushering another new life into the world.

He should go home.

But was it worth it? It wasn't just the travel time, including quite a long walk to the staff parking area. He hadn't unpacked anything in the apartment he'd taken on a short-term lease before he'd decided the priority should be to sort out his office. There was no linen on his bed or towels in the bathroom. He might be able to unearth a mug but he hadn't been to a supermarket yet either, so there was no coffee or milk in the fridge. This was, in fact, one of the very rare occasions when he had to wonder if work should always take priority over his personal life.

'It's Mr Smythe, isn't it?' The ward receptionist looked away from the computer screen in front of her. 'Can I help with anything?'

He read her name badge. 'Thanks, Rita,' he said. 'And please call me Lachlan. Tell me, what's the morning traffic like these days, coming here from Notting Hill? I've been away from London for a few years now.'

Rita looked to be in her fifties and had a welcoming, motherly vibe that was no doubt much appreciated by stressed young couples arriving to face a major event in their lives. She wasn't looking very reassuring now, however.

'Awful,' she said. 'It would take you a good thirty minutes at this time of night with no real traffic and in rush hour…goodness me, I'd be leaving at least an hour before I wanted to be here. Ninety minutes, even.'

'I thought that might be the case. Maybe I'll just stay here and find some coffee or a comfortable chair for a snooze. I'd rather like an early start and to be here for the shift changeover. Great way to get the feel of a new hospital.'

'We do have some on-call bedrooms near the staffroom, if you want to be really comfortable—on the other side of the corridor where your office is. They get booked by the registrars on call but I could check to see if there are any available?'

'Thanks, but I have a splinter skill I learned as a junior doctor of being able to sleep just about anywhere for short periods of time. If I can find a hot shower later, I'll survive until day's end.' He smiled at Rita. 'It's my own fault. I should have been home many hours ago.'

'Just as well you weren't, from what I heard,' Rita said. She smiled back at him. 'Welcome to Queen Mary's, Lachlan. You know how to make an entrance, that's for sure. There are some nice squashy armchairs in the staffroom. I've fallen asleep in them myself at times. The coffee's not bad and there's always plenty of toast. The showers in the locker rooms are good. At least they are on the women's side. Can't say I've tested the men's showers.'

'I'll let you know, for future reference.' Lachlan turned away, laughing. 'I'll go and find some of that coffee. And toast. I've just realised I forgot to have any dinner. Oh…if you see Pippa and she's got a free minute, can you tell her where I am? I'd like to talk to her.'

'He wants to talk to me?' Pippa had just written BORN across the status box on the whiteboard for Room Six. She turned to frown at Rita. 'Why?'

'He didn't say. But he did say that he was living in Notting Hill.' Rita raised her eyebrows. 'That's rather posh, isn't it?'

'People might say that about me, living in central Richmond, but I can assure you that my rented cottage that's about the same size as a postage stamp is very far from posh. What else did he say?'

'That he wasn't going home. He's going to stay here and eat toast and drink coffee and then have a shower and be here for the shift changeover at seven-thirty a.m.' Rita blew out a breath. 'Have you ever met a new consultant who's quite so… hands-on?'

'No…but at least he seems to know what he's doing.' Pippa had an image of those hands right now. Moving confidently and swiftly to perform the fine motor skills of using a single finger to occlude a vein at the same time as removing a needle from a cannula, screwing a plug into place and attaching the tubing of an IV giving set.

'I am overdue for a break,' she added. 'Guess I could go and have a coffee and see what he wants to talk to me about. You'll know where I am if anyone needs me.'

Pippa hoped her sudden nervousness wasn't showing. She could feel her heart racing and it felt like an effort to suck in a new breath. Had she done something wrong earlier? Maybe she had underestimated how boggy Helen's uterus had been post-delivery but she hadn't been bleeding unduly and it hadn't been painful to have her tummy massaged. It had definitely begun contracting before she'd left her alone in the room.

Her heart sank like a stone at the sudden thought that he might, instead, want to tell her that Helen's condition had deteriorated again and that baby Jack was in danger of losing his mother.

No…she might have only met this man a few hours ago but she was absolutely certain that if he had any involvement at all with a patient who was in trouble he wouldn't be in the staffroom drinking coffee and eating toast.

The thought of toast made a knot form in her stomach. Or was that due to her nerves? She didn't think she'd done anything wrong. She'd delivered two healthy babies. Helen's emergency had been successfully dealt with without her needing to go to Theatre. Stella was peacefully asleep now and it looked as if the scare she'd had for her pregnancy might be over.

Maybe she was nervous for a reason that had nothing to do with anything professional. There was something about this man that was…a little unsettling, that was what it was.

Or… Pippa stifled a yawn. Perhaps she was just tired. And hungry.

At three-thirty a.m. she would have expected to find a few weary-looking staff members taking a break, but the only person in the room was Lachlan. He had a newspaper open in front of him on the central table and he put down a half-empty cup of coffee with a grimace.

'Coffee's great when it's hot,' he said. 'And revolting when it's cold.' He smiled at Pippa. 'That'll teach me for getting stuck on a crossword puzzle.'

Oh, my…

That was a real smile. One that reached his eyes enough to crinkle the corners. Eyes that were almost as dark as her own, but they weren't brown. Even in this light, she could see that they were blue. His hair was brown, though. Brown and wavy and soft looking.

He wasn't just attractive, she realised. He was…absolutely gorgeous.

And that knot in her stomach had just sent off

a volley of sparks that were travelling through her body at the speed of light. Oh, help…*she* was attracted to him.

Hastily, she looked away. She stepped away even, heading for the bench.

'Rita said you wanted to talk to me?'

He sounded as if he was still smiling. 'I did. I just wanted to tell you how well you managed that emergency with Helen. If the other staff members in this department are half as good at their jobs as you are, I'm going to enjoy working here very much.'

'Oh…' Pippa could feel her cheeks going pink, which was never the best look for a redhead. 'Thank you.' She felt too shy to tell him that she'd been just as impressed with him. 'I'm going to make myself a cup of coffee,' she said instead. 'I can top yours up for you if you like?'

'It's okay. I suspect I've had more than enough caffeine.'

Pippa opened the bag of sliced white bread on the bench and then went to the fridge to get out some butter and a block of cheese. She flicked on the sandwich maker.

'Can I interest you in a cheese toastie instead?'

'Now you're talking…'

Oh-h… The approval in his voice was a verbal caress. Pippa took extra care to butter the bread right to the edges and fill the sandwich with extra cheese so it would turn out to be crispy and brown and irresistibly delicious. She wanted to give him that pleasure. And she wanted to see the expression on his face when he took that first bite.

She closed the top of the sandwich maker and clipped it shut. It might be a good idea to shut off the direction her thoughts wanted to go in as well.

'Have you had an update on Helen?' she asked.

'She's doing well. No signs of any further excessive bleeding, but they'll keep her in ICU until they're sure she's not going to have any complications from the aggressive fluid replacement. Terry's with her. Jack's being looked after in the special care baby unit but he's fine.'

Pippa risked a sideways glance. She couldn't help it when she could hear the smile in his voice again. She wanted to see it as well.

'They've got you to thank for a happy outcome,' Lachlan said quietly. 'If she'd been left much longer with a bleed like that, it could have been a very different story, so thank you.'

'I think the fact that you were still in the building was what made the real difference,' Pippa said. 'I have to say I was very surprised to see you come through the door. And relieved, I have to confess. It was a scary situation.'

'Intense,' Lachlan agreed. 'Bit of a trial by fire in getting to know a new colleague, yes?'

'Yes…' Pippa lifted the fragrant toastie from the machine to a plate and opened a drawer to find a knife. 'Speaking of fire, we'll need to wait a few minutes to eat this. It'll be like molten lava in the middle.'

'Good. Maybe you can help me with the crossword clue I'm stuck on while we wait.'

'Sure.' Pippa sat down opposite him. 'Shoot.'

'Six letters, a U in the middle and a D at the end. Clue is "Succinct description of an old woman who lived in a form of footwear".'

'The one who lived in a shoe? Who had so many children she didn't know what to do?'

'That's the one.'

Pippa laughed. 'Stupid?' she suggested.

She was still laughing as she watched the smile on his face turning into a grin and then heard his own rumble of laughter. It was a rather delicious sound.

Even better, *she'd* made him laugh. How good was that?

Too good.

She could feel those sparks again. Not just in her body—it felt as if the air was thick with them. They were settling on her skin and getting caught in her hair. She was breathing them in. She could taste them on her tongue and they were just as delicious as the sound of his laughter.

The strident sound of her pager beeping had never been so welcome.

Lachlan Smythe was her new boss. He might not be wearing a ring but that was no guarantee he was single.

Two red flags.

He was also a *doctor*, for heaven's sake.

Pippa should know better.

She *did* know better.

'Gotta go,' she said, reading her pager. 'New human arriving.'

'But you haven't had any of your sandwich.'

'It's all yours.' Pippa was on her feet and turning towards the door. The sooner she put some distance between herself and Lachlan, the better. 'Consider it a welcome gift. Enjoy…'

She walked away without looking back.

CHAPTER THREE

FECUND.

The answer to that crossword clue should have been instantly obvious to an obstetrician.

But, deep down, he was delighted that he'd missed it. Because Philippa Gordon—he'd learnt her full name in a departmental meeting this afternoon—had made him laugh.

He liked her.

He really liked her.

But beneath that humour was something that felt even more of a connection. Wasn't there a proverb about many a true word being spoken in jest? Was Pippa, like him, working with babies because she loved them but she didn't want—or couldn't have—her own?

Whatever.

It was none of his business.

He hadn't seen her since the day shift had come on board after the night of that dramatic post-partum haemorrhage and she'd gone home for some well-deserved sleep, and he hadn't given her a second thought throughout the busyness of his first official day as the new head of obstetrics at The Queen Mary.

He found himself thinking about her again that evening, however, when he was finally in his apartment, making up his bed. Counting down the minutes until his head could hit the pillow because he was quite ready to sleep the clock around after such a full-on start to his new position.

A trial by fire, indeed, as he'd said to Pippa.

And that was kind of an appropriate turn of phrase, given the colour of her hair. Long hair. Tightly wound into a braid. What did it look like when it was unravelled? Was it straight or wavy? He was sure it would feel soft. Silky…

Lachlan shook his head as if it would be enough to shake off a disturbingly inappropriate direction for his thoughts to be going in. He went into his bathroom and turned the shower on. Briefly, he considered turning the temperature control to cold in the hope that this could be doused.

This…*attraction*.

It had been there from the first moment he'd laid eyes on her. It had been simmering in the background and easily ignored when he'd been working so closely with her but…oh, man… when she'd made him laugh, it had suddenly exploded into something that was new territory for Lachlan. He'd never been this attracted, this quickly, to anyone since he'd been a teenager and hadn't yet learned that it was better for everybody involved to keep a tight control of that kind of thing. Otherwise, you were playing with fire, and it was inevitable that someone would get burned.

Thoughts of flames seemed to be a recurring theme around this woman and Lachlan thought he knew why. It was because the heat they produced could be dangerous unless very well controlled and Lachlan's interactions with women were always very well controlled. It wasn't that he didn't enjoy female company or appreciate having a healthy sex life. Not at all! He loved women as much as he loved babies. He enjoyed the familiar sensations of a physical attraction and the building of a friendship that could include the pleasure of sex. Under controlled conditions, of course. There were boundaries that would never be crossed and if that wasn't understood and accepted right from the start then the attraction would never go any further.

But this felt different.

So different, it was like nothing Lachlan had ever experienced before.

This one was fierce enough to be a warning

he couldn't ignore and he would be well advised to back away.

Fast.

Heads of departments didn't do Queen Mary's twelve-hour night shifts that ran from seven-thirty p.m. to seven-thirty a.m. so it was no surprise that Pippa's path did not cross with that of Lachlan Smythe for the rest of that week.

It should have made it so much easier to deal with that unusual level of attraction to a man she'd only just met and knew nothing about. Her boss, no less. She needed to parcel it up and put it where it belonged—well away from her professional life. Given that it was a strong enough feeling to make a shiny thing she would be better not to even consider playing with, she needed to keep it away from her personal life as well.

It was making it far less easy that she continued to be too aware of his appearance in her world and to be learning things about him despite not having sought the information. The hospital grapevine was humming with reports of the most recent senior appointment. Conclusions were being drawn and opinions whispered and Pippa had heard far too many of them for comfort. It was impossible not to hear them on a quieter night shift.

Have you seen the new HoD of Obstetrics? Phew...he's a bit of all right, isn't he?

Someone who's seen his CV says he's single, but he's forty years old so he must be divorced. Nobody's heard of an ex-wife, though. Or any kids.

Maybe he's gay.

He was born and bred in London but he's got seriously itchy feet. He's lived in the USA, Australia, Canada and Switzerland.

He got into ocean swimming in Australia to keep fit. He's been asking about good places to go wild swimming around London.

Wild? As in naked? Hahaha... I'm in...

He's very, very good at his job. He hadn't even officially started work here but he virtually single-handedly saved the life of a first-time mother who could have bled out.

That snippet had made Pippa shake her head. Not that she was about to add her two cents' worth and remind people that she had been there as well, along with a cast of many others, including some unseen but crucial staff members in places like the blood bank.

But others had made her curious.

Why was he single?

Why did he keep moving? Not just hospitals or cities but whole countries? Continents, even. Was he running away from something? Or some*one*?

And…*did* he ever swim naked?

By the time she'd finished the week on nights that, fortunately, she didn't need to do very often, the grapevine had the new topic of a juicy scandal involving a married cardiologist and a young technician from the catheter laboratory. Pippa made a considerable effort to ignore any details about that development and the unwelcome trips down memory lane they could push her into, but on day shifts there was far more distraction available and it was relatively easy to avoid company in the staffroom or cafeteria, where that kind of gossip was most likely to be shared.

Maybe she should have tried harder to avoid the information she seemed to have gathered about Lachlan Smythe, but that was partly human nature at work, wasn't it? Toying with attraction was more than pleasant. Her personal memory lane was rather too full of painful potholes. It was so much easier to swerve the prospect of pain than deny yourself a flash of pleasure.

While it would be relatively simple to avoid gossip during a day shift, Pippa knew it would be more likely that she would have to interact with their new HoD. There were complications in childbirth that demanded the attention of someone more highly qualified than she was as a midwife. An awkward presentation, perhaps, or a multiple birth or a baby in distress. An instrumental or surgical delivery was always in the hands of an obstetrician and, of course, there were ward rounds, outpatient clinics and just… being in the same workspace.

Pippa was, however, confident that the odds of Lachlan being the senior staff member she worked with more than any others were low and, even if she did find herself working in close proximity to him, she was just as confident that any personal attraction would not undermine her ability to do her job well. That the winds of fate were providing a test for her resolve on her first morning back on day shift was a little disconcerting but it was a good thing, Pippa decided, as she began to prepare a nervous woman for an elective C-section on the only day of the week that Mr Smythe had a full theatre list.

She would start as she intended to continue.

Completely focused.

Without revealing the slightest hint that there could be any less than professional thoughts in her head. Hopefully, those weird sparks would have burned themselves out by now.

It would be no different than it was to work with the anaesthetist, Peter, who came in to administer the spinal anaesthetic.

'So this is Kate Mulligan,' she told him, turning the wrist ID for Peter to check for himself. 'She's thirty-two and is thirty-eight weeks pregnant. She's in for an elective C-section this morning due to a Grade Two placenta previa that has a margin of less than two centimetres from the cervical os.'

'Hi, Kate, I'm Peter. I'll be giving you your spinal anaesthetic and looking after you in Theatre. How are you feeling this morning?'

'Terrified,' Kate admitted.

'I can give you something to help with that,' Peter said. He smiled at Pippa. 'Can you draw up a dose of midazolam for me, please? We'll let that take effect before we get started.'

Pippa had worked with Peter on many occasions over the years she'd been at Queen Mary's. He was a perfectly nice guy but there had never been any sparks between them. She would channel this feeling of professional ease when she got to Theatre.

She supported Kate as the cannula was inserted into her back and the medication delivered to provide complete anaesthesia from the waist down. She helped her into a theatre gown, took off her nail polish and put tape over the rings she was wearing. She took another set of vital signs on Kate and printed a strip of the CTG recording on her baby.

'You're going to meet your daughter very soon,' she said. 'How exciting is that?'

It was Pippa's job to take the CTG machine up to Theatre and go through the pre-operative checklist with the theatre staff. Both Kate's husband and Pippa needed to get dressed to be in the operating room during the surgery. Covered from the hat over her hair to the disposable booties on her feet, Pippa suddenly felt almost as relaxed as Kate was, thanks to her medication. She was completely disguised. The surgeon about to come in from the scrub room would probably not even recognise her, especially as she stood back then, with no further responsibilities until the baby was delivered and handed into her care.

That feeling of protection lasted as Lachlan came in with his registrar, chatted to Kate for a moment, on the other side of the drapes pinned up as a screen, and then positioned himself to begin the surgery.

'All set?' He actually had the scalpel in his hand and was poised to make the first incision as his glance raked the staff around him.

Pippa could hear the murmur of assent but didn't make a sound herself. Lachlan's gaze had only grazed hers for a microsecond but she knew he had not only recognised her, he was pleased to see her.

And dammit…she had to stand here, outside

of the sterile field, and feel the sparkle that was still there. Increased, if anything, by observing not only Lachlan's surgical skills but the way he interacted with both his team and his patient.

'Are you ready, Kate? We're going to take the drapes down so you can see your baby being born.'

'I…think so… I won't be able to see too much though, will I?'

'No. Your tummy is hiding all the gruesome bits, I promise. I'm going to lift her out and, if she doesn't need any extra help, we'll put her straight onto your chest and wait a minute or two to cut the cord. Okay?'

Kate's response was more like a sob. 'Okay…'

Pippa was standing close now, with a sterile towel across her hands. If the baby needed resuscitation, she would be put onto the towel rather than going straight to the skin-to-skin contact with her mother. Pippa would take her to the heated cocoon of the resuscitation unit to one side of the room, to do the first Apgar score and get her dry and warm. They had a paediatrician on standby if they were needed.

But this baby opened her mouth and gave her first cry the moment she was eased out of the womb. Lachlan handled the slippery little bundle with great care as the nurses lowered the drapes and he carried the baby to lay her gently onto Kate's chest. Pippa stepped in so that she could cover the baby with a towel to help keep her warm and do the first Apgar score and for just for a heartbeat, as he lowered the baby, her gaze caught Lachlan's. Being so much closer this time, she could see the crinkles at the corners of his eyes and the warmth that made them such an incredibly dark blue.

He was happy, she realised. Not because someone had made him laugh this time, but because he was holding a new, precious baby in his hands that he'd helped arrive safely in the world. She knew that happiness. It filled her own heart every time. It was the best of moments and it was what had kept her in this job because it never failed to balance the worst of moments, even if it couldn't eliminate them.

This connection, on what was both a professional and personal level, was exactly what Pippa had needed. It made the nuisance of navigating unwanted sparks worthwhile. She could respect this man. Even better, she could appreciate working with him instead of hoping to avoid it and, on a purely instinctive level, she was quite sure that she could trust him.

It should have worn off by now.

Lachlan had been in his new job for nearly three weeks now. He could find his way around

The Queen Mary with no difficulties at all. He was familiar with most of his new colleagues and quite comfortable running his departmental meetings and liaising with other Heads of Departments. He was enjoying the clinical work and loving being back in his hometown. So much so that he was stopping on his way home to have a look at a property on the market in Richmond because he was already sick of getting stuck in rush-hour traffic at both ends of his working days.

It was the only real fly in the ointment of this decision to come back to the UK.

Although he was also slightly disappointed that ignoring the unusual level of attraction he felt towards Pippa Gordon wasn't making it vanish as quickly as he'd anticipated.

It didn't help that he seemed to see her more often than any of the other midwives who worked in and around the birthing suite. And he didn't just see her. He worked with her. A lot. How was it that she seemed to be present almost every time he did a C-section—elective or emergent? And yes, as such an experienced midwife, she was going to be given the more high-risk mothers to care for, but she seemed to get more than her share of births that needed obstetrical assistance. He'd even spoken to her in the outpatient department this afternoon.

Okay…that had been his choice. But he'd known she was working in the antenatal clinic and that she'd want to know the results of the latest reassurance scan on Stella.

'Her Braxton Hicks contractions have settled to completely normal levels and everything else is looking good. She's still a bit anxious, but getting past the twenty-four-week mark and knowing that the baby is viable has been a real boost.'

'I know, I saw her in the waiting room. She's so much happier. Getting well past the stage that she had lost her first baby has been a big help. She's not going to stop being anxious, but she did say that she was going to go and buy a Moses basket when she gets to twenty-eight weeks and I know what a big deal that is for her.'

'She mentioned you in her appointment with me. Said that you were the best possible person who could have looked after her that night she got admitted. That you really seemed to understand what she was going through.'

Pippa seemed to appreciate the feedback. They'd shared a smile, nothing more.

It had been a purely professional interaction. So why was he thinking of her as he headed away from work? And when the attractive estate agent was giving him signals of being interested in more than selling him this property?

'It's a stunning property,' he told her.

It was. A detached Edwardian house that was almost spitting distance to Marble Hill Park, with an upstairs view across the Thames to the huge expanse of Richmond Park.

'I think four bedrooms might be a little too big for me, though,' he added.

Why was he even looking at a family home?

Especially one that had a view to Richmond Park. He'd learned to ride his bike on the green spaces and pathways of that park. He'd helped his beloved younger brother Liam to get good enough to ditch his training wheels before he even started school.

Before the first signs of possibly the most heartbreaking type of the hereditary disease of Huntington's—the rare juvenile form that would slowly but inexorably destroy and then finally take his life when he was only fifteen.

But the tragedy of the disease and how it had affected the whole family hadn't been the first thing he'd thought of when he'd noticed the view, had it? It had been a happy memory of racing each other on their bikes. Of the triumphant smile on Liam's face when Lachlan had let him win. Of the family picnic they'd been having that day. While still incredibly poignant, he could feel the notes of joy in that memory and that was…priceless.

He'd only been half-listening to what the estate agent was saying about getting a feel for the market and how this was the most exceptional property she'd seen in a long time.

'I'll contact you if anything smaller comes up for sale,' she said finally. 'Check out the area while you're here, though. It's got a lot going for it. There's a fabulous pub just a few blocks away. And a shopping precinct that's got a good supermarket.'

Lachlan did check it out. Not the pub, but he did need some groceries and the local supermarket was one he liked for its ready-made meals that only needed a few minutes in the microwave to taste like home cooking.

He was heading from the frozen food section to the checkout when he rounded a corner and came too close to crashing his trolley into someone else's.

'I'm so sorry,' he said. 'I wasn't paying attention.'

'That's not like you.'

His head jerked up at hearing a voice he recognised instantly.

'Pippa! What on earth are you doing here?'

She was smiling at him. 'Exactly what *you're* doing. Except...' She glanced into his trolley. 'I do tend to buy things that need cooking.'

Yes. Her trolley was full of fresh vegetables like tomatoes and garlic and spinach. She had fresh pasta as well. Olive oil and Parmesan cheese.

Lachlan was a big fan of Italian food.

She was wearing jeans. And a top that was a pretty shade of yellow. And her hair was loose, flowing down her back like a silky curtain. It was straight.

Lachlan was a big fan of straight, silky hair. Especially when it was hanging loose.

'And I live around here,' Pippa added. 'I thought you lived in Notting Hill?'

'How did you know that?'

'Ah…'

Lachlan saw the pink flush in her cheeks. Why was she embarrassed? Because she'd obviously been talking about him?

Because…she was also feeling that static electricity sensation that happened to him whenever he was too close to her?

It was stronger than ever right now. Because they weren't at work. This wasn't, in any way, a professional encounter but he didn't want it to become awkward.

'I was looking at a house for sale,' he told her. 'I'm hoping to live a bit closer to work myself. The estate agent told me to check the area out on my way home. She said there's a great pub nearby.'

'The one on the other side of the supermarket car park? The White Swan?'

'That's the one. Is it as good as I'm told?'

'I've never been.' Pippa shrugged. 'I don't tend to go into pubs by myself.'

She was by herself? *Single?*

'Neither do I,' he said.

Lachlan could hear a voice in the back of his head.

No... Don't do it. Do. Not. Do. It.

He ignored the directive.

'You wouldn't have the time to pop in with me now, by any chance, would you? That would mean we could both find out whether it's any good without looking like dodgy characters who like to drink alone.'

His invitation hung in the air between them for a split second. Long enough for Lachlan to wish he'd kept his mouth shut. Oh, help...did Pippa think he was hitting on her?

Was he hitting on her?

He was just about to open his mouth again and give them both an easy way out by telling her he'd actually remembered a prior engagement, but she beat him to saying anything.

'Why not?' Her tone made it a perfectly reasonable suggestion. One with no strings attached. 'I've always wondered what it's like inside.'

Lachlan had lost the slightest inclination to withdraw his suggestion. He was, in fact, feeling delighted. He didn't care that his smile probably looked more like a grin.

'I'll meet you on the other side of the checkout.'

CHAPTER FOUR

IT WAS EVERYTHING you could want in a traditional English pub.

Hanging baskets full of bright flowers outside, the gleam of polished wood on the bar and tables inside. Old copper pots, kettles and vintage lanterns dangled from the beams and there were horse brasses and faded oil paintings on the walls.

It was cluttered and cosy and comfortable. Popular enough in this after work time slot for the available seating to look limited.

Lachlan let go of the heavy door he'd held open for Pippa. 'Why don't you see if you can find us a seat?' he suggested. 'What can I get you to drink?'

Pippa met his gaze. She wasn't sure she should be here at all, let alone having a drink with her new boss. This was starting to feel too much like a date. But that tingle in her gut was telling her that she would be an idiot to walk away, so she shrugged instead.

'Ah, why not?' she said. 'I'm walking home. A glass of prosecco would be lovely.'

'I might join you.' Lachlan grinned. 'Just for one. Although, with the traffic out there, I won't be driving any more than a walking pace, anyway.'

Pippa moved off as she spotted people getting up to leave a table near the fireplace. Not that it was cold enough to warrant an open fire, but the flicker of flames certainly added to the welcoming ambience. It also made her think of that warning not to play with fire.

Was that what she was doing, spending time with Lachlan that had nothing to do with anything professional?

He didn't seem to be worried about it. 'This is nice,' he said as he came to the table with two flutes of fizzy wine. 'It's a long time since I've been in a pub. Or even out with a colleague. I have a bad habit of making friends and then changing jobs and countries and leaving them all behind.'

Was he thinking he might become friends with her?

Would she want to be friends with him?

It was worth consideration. Being friends, with the definite boundaries that automatically imposed, might defuse an attraction that could be a nuisance. Or would spending time with him like this make it worse? It didn't seem to be having that effect right now. Pippa was interested in learning more about him, not imagining what it might be like to be kissed by him.

Well…okay…maybe that *was* hovering in the back of her mind.

She hastily lifted her glass for a first sip of her wine.

'I did hear that you moved around a lot,' she said. 'Where were you before you came to Queen Mary's? Somewhere in the States?'

'Johns Hopkins. In Baltimore, Maryland. It's a general hospital that's got a great focus on teaching and research.'

'It's one of the world's most famous hospitals. I have heard of it.' Pippa laughed. 'I've heard of Washington DC as well. That's part of Maryland, isn't it?'

'Next door neighbour. DC stands for District of Colombia. It's not a state and doesn't belong to any state. Cool place to visit. Have you been there?'

'I haven't been out of the UK in years. Haven't changed my job, either. Maybe I'm not as adventurous as you are.'

'I love new challenges,' Lachlan admitted. 'And fresh starts. Arriving somewhere with no baggage, other than what I put my clothes and books in.'

'So you travel alone?' Pippa hastily reached for her glass to take another sip of her drink. That was a rather personal question, wasn't it? She risked a quick glance and found that he was watching her.

'Always.' He lifted an eyebrow. 'How 'bout you?'

'If I was going to travel it would definitely be alone,' she agreed.

Lachlan's other eyebrow rose as well. 'You sound very sure about that.'

'I'm sure about many things.'

Lachlan laughed. 'Good for you.'

It was the second time she'd made him laugh and it felt even better than the first time. This was like a compliment—as if he approved of her being so sure of her own mind.

'So you live around here?'

'How did you know that?' She was deliberately repeating the question he'd disarmed her with earlier, but the curl of his mouth told her he knew exactly what she was doing and he wasn't remotely embarrassed.

'Because you told me you were walking,' he reminded her. 'And in the supermarket I do believe you said "I live around here".' His eyebrows rose and his glance was suddenly noticeably more intense. 'How did you know where *I* lived?'

'The grapevine,' she muttered. 'Not that I normally pay any attention to gossip but…you did create a bit of a buzz when you arrived. Especially after riding in on your white horse and saving a life before you were even officially on duty.'

'*We* saved a life,' he said firmly. He took a longer sip of wine. 'So…what else were people saying about me?'

'Only good stuff. How well respected you are in your field. Some people wondered what made you come back here. Especially to Richmond, when you could have got a job at another world-famous hospital like Guy's or Great Ormond Street.'

'I grew up here,' Lachlan told her. 'Learned to ride a bike in Richmond Park. Were they saying anything else I should know about?'

Pippa had had just enough wine to make her feel ever so slightly mischievous. 'I did pick up on the rumour that you didn't seem to have a wife. Or kids.'

Lachlan's face stilled and Pippa would have decided that she'd overstepped a boundary but his gaze was steady.

'No,' he said. He held her gaze even longer. 'How 'bout you?'

'No,' she replied, using the same tone he had—as if it was no big deal or wasn't up for discussion. But then she felt guilty because she'd been the one to step onto such personal ground. 'Been there, done that,' she said. 'Wouldn't recommend it.'

'You've been married?'

'Just the once.' It was time to lighten the atmosphere, Pippa decided. 'He decided to upgrade.' She kept her tone and expression deadpan. 'To an obstetrician.'

Lachlan grimaced. 'I apologise on behalf of my specialty,' he said.

Pippa snorted. 'He was a cardiologist.'

Lachlan was just as deadpan as she had been. 'In that case, I apologise on behalf of my gender. Possibly all of mankind.'

It was genuine laughter this time and Pippa remembered just how sexy it was for a man to be able to make you laugh.

They both sat in a companionable silence then, finishing their drinks. It was Lachlan who broke it.

'This really has been nice,' he said.

'It has,' Pippa agreed. Too nice. Lachlan was intelligent, easy on the eye, easy to talk to and he'd made her laugh. What more could any girl ask for?

'Can we do it again some time?'

It was Pippa who caught and held *his* gaze this

time and she knew it was a very direct look. She had felt the muscles around her eyes emphasising the focus. She might as well have had a speech bubble above her head like a cartoon character.

'I'm not hitting on you,' he said. 'I like your company and…' if she wasn't mistaken, there was a mischievous glint in his eyes now '… I'm the new boy at school, you know? It's good to make friends.'

Pippa shook her head but she was smiling. Lachlan dropped his gaze to the bags of groceries she had beside her chair.

'Are you sure you want to walk? I could give you a lift.'

'I'm sure,' Pippa said. She got to her feet and bent to pick up the bags. 'Thanks for the drink, Lachlan. Maybe I'll see you at work tomorrow?'

'You will. And you're welcome. You didn't answer my question, though.'

Pippa's expression was intended to suggest careful thought. 'I'll check the rule book,' she said. 'Just in case there's some fine print about drinking prosecco with your boss.'

'You have a rule book?'

'Of course. Don't you?'

'Are we talking professional or personal?'

'Both,' Pippa said. 'And in this instance the rules could be in two different sections.'

The way Lachlan lifted his eyebrows was a mix of surprise and genuine interest. 'Which are?'

'Professional relationships,' Pippa said. 'And… dating.'

'Ah…'

Oh, help…why had she got carried away enough with this idea of a rule book that she'd said that out loud? Now they were both thinking of being in each other's company when it could be more than simply two colleagues bumping into each other away from work.

And for her, at least, the prospect was a little too enticing for comfort. Pippa turned away with a shake of her head, as if she was dismissing an inappropriate suggestion.

But she could hear him speaking quietly behind her as she walked away.

'It's your book,' he said. 'And I get the feeling that it's you that makes the rules.'

The knowledge that Pippa Gordon's husband had left her for another woman was a snippet of gossip that Lachlan would have ignored if he'd heard it from anyone else. He might not have even believed it, in fact. For heaven's sake, the woman was gorgeous. Competent. Funny. And she could, presumably, cook Italian food. What had the guy been thinking?

He found himself wondering how long they had been married for. Long enough for her to be so devastated she had no intention of trying the state of matrimony ever again, anyway. She must have been very deeply in love, Lachlan decided.

Weirdly, even though he had no intention of ever getting married himself, he felt jealous of the guy.

He hadn't been averse to marriage.

And Pippa had chosen him.

He only saw her in passing the next day, but there was something different about the way she smiled after they exchanged greetings.

They had met each other outside of work hours and their shared workspace, which had opened a door into something different, and spending even a short time together had been…nice.

Very nice.

They had a great basis for friendship. A connection in a shared career that would never leave them short of something interesting to talk about but, more importantly, they had made each other laugh about things that had nothing to do with work. About that stupid crossword clue and him offering an apology on behalf of every person on earth that shared his gender.

He loved having made her laugh.

It wasn't that often that someone made him laugh with such genuine amusement.

Didn't that make them halfway to being friends already?

Lachlan hoped so. He thoroughly enjoyed the company of women and it was very hard to have a genuine friendship with someone of the opposite sex without courting expectations.

He liked Pippa. He liked that she was confident enough to make her own rules.

He had his own rules about relationships and dating that were clearly stricter than Pippa's, given that she had been married, but he'd like to hear more about hers and ask which ones she found worked especially well. Who wasn't up for a bit of self-improvement, after all?

He didn't ask, of course. But he did appreciate the occasions their paths crossed, even if it was simply in the corridor or an outpatient clinic. Working together in Theatre or on the ward was a bonus.

He liked the way she was with the women she was supporting in labour—encouraging and appreciative of their efforts, she knew how far to push them but also had a good instinct for a woman or baby who was getting into difficulties. He had only been working here for a short time but he knew that if it was Pippa calling for assistance it was very unlikely to be a false alarm.

Not that he immediately knew it was Pippa when he responded to an alarm in Room One, having gone past the reception area to check his pigeonhole for mail on the way back to his office from a meeting. He walked into the room to find a woman kneeling on the bed, the midwife hidden behind her. He recognised Pippa's voice the instant she continued with her instructions.

'Put your head right down on the bed, Ashley—that's it. Bum up in the air as high as you can. That's great…'

'What's happening?' The man standing near the window was looking confused. 'I don't understand. I thought it was a good thing when the waters broke.'

Lachlan knew exactly what was happening. He went to pull gloves from the box on the wall. 'Cord prolapse?' he queried tersely. It was the obvious reason to put a woman into a position where gravity could help take the pressure off an umbilical cord that had come out in front of the presenting part of a baby.

'Yes.' Pippa's face appeared as she straightened to move to the end of the bed. She was also donning a fresh pair of gloves. 'The waters broke about two minutes ago when I put the CTG on to monitor the heart rate and contractions. Some meconium. It's been a long second stage. Cord prolapse was visible. And pulsatile.'

Pulsatile was good. It meant the baby was still alive. The priority was to keep pressure off the cord until they could deliver this baby, which needed to happen as quickly as possible.

Another midwife came through the door in response to the alarm. 'Get Theatre on standby, please,' Lachlan told her. 'And get a paeds team on standby too.'

The CTG straps were still around Ashley's belly and he could see that the baby's heart rate was slower than he would have liked.

So could Pippa. 'You're going to feel me putting my hand inside,' she told Ashley. 'I'm going to be pushing on baby's head, just gently.'

'Why? *Ow...* Why do you need to do that?'

'To stop baby's head pressing on the cord,' Lachlan explained, stepping closer. 'What was the last heart rate you recorded, Pippa—before the cord prolapse?'

'One forty.'

'It's back to one twenty now. Up from ninety-four.'

'Good. I'll switch to external supra-pubic pressure as soon as I'm sure the head is above the pelvic rim.'

'I want to push,' Ashley groaned.

'*No*. Don't push,' Pippa said urgently. 'Not yet.' She looked up at Lachlan. 'She's fully dilated,' she told him. 'And I can feel that the cord's still pulsatile.'

She held his gaze, knowing exactly what he

was weighing up. It was possible that a vaginal delivery could be quicker than a Caesarean but it would require a team effort from the mother, the midwife and an experienced obstetrician. Lachlan might have been more reluctant to consider it if he didn't have this much faith in Pippa.

'Any contra-indications to an expedited delivery?'

'She's tired,' Pippa said. 'But she'll give it everything she's got.'

'Forceps kit?'

'On the trolley. There's a gown there, too.'

'Ashley? Do you still feel ready to push?'

'Yes.' The word was a sob.

'Okay. We're going to wait for your next contraction and then I'm going to let go of baby's head and help you turn onto your back. We're going to need your baby to be born as fast as possible so you are really going to have to push hard. I'm going to help as much as I can and Lachlan is going to help with forceps, but you've got an important job to do.'

'I can do it…' Ashley was breathing hard. 'I want to do it. Ooh… I can feel another contraction starting…'

Pippa looked up at Lachlan, who was shoving his arms into the gown a midwife was holding for him. He held her gaze and then gave a single nod before glancing up at the clock.

'Let's go,' he said.

Pippa's hand was aching and badly cramped by the time she could release the pressure she'd been putting on the baby's head. She also glanced up at the clock as she helped Ashley turn onto her back. They had a limited time frame to get this baby out because its oxygen supply was going to be compromised as soon as Ashley started pushing the baby's head down, which would press the cord against the pelvic bones and prevent the movement of life-sustaining oxygen. If they couldn't get the baby delivered in time, it would be fatal.

'Push…' Pippa encouraged Ashley. 'Push, push, *push*. Keep it going… That's it… Don't stop… Push again…'

She glanced up at Lachlan, now gowned, gloved and masked and looking every inch the surgeon he was. He had to be as aware of the tension in this room as Pippa was but he gave the impression of being completely calm and in control. More staff members were in the room now and a nurse was helping with the medical equipment on the trolley, unrolling a sterile kit that had the forceps Lachlan was going to use to help this delivery happen swiftly. He lubricated the first blade and kept his hand across the back of it to protect Ashely as he slid it into place. With the second blade in place, he locked them together and positioned his hands, ready to provide gentle traction to augment Ashley's next push. He gave Pippa a tiny nod.

'I need you to push again,' Pippa told her. 'Even if the contraction is wearing off. Take a big breath and push down…as hard as you can.'

Ashley was still gasping from her efforts. 'I *can't*…'

'Yes, you can, sweetheart.' Pippa's voice was calm. Confident. 'You're doing *so* well. One more push…as hard as you can. That's the way. *Push*…'

'I can see it.' Ashley's partner sounded awed. 'Our baby's coming, Ash…'

The baby slid out, looking completely limp. They needed to move fast. Pippa grabbed a warmed sterile towel as Lachlan clamped and cut the cord. He took the suction bulb from the midwife and cleared the airway of the infant. Pippa briskly but gently dried the baby but the stimulation wasn't enough to start it breathing. She put another towel across her hands and Lachlan lifted the tiny body and put it onto the towel. Pippa turned and took it to the resuscitation unit at one side of the room, where they could keep the baby warm. The paediatric team hadn't arrived yet so it was up to her and Lachlan to resuscitate this baby boy.

'Why isn't he crying?' Ashley was trying to sit up. 'What's happening? Is he going to be all right?'

Her partner was watching in horror. The other midwife was moving in to support them both.

Pippa knew where everything they needed was kept in the drawers of the unit. She handed a stethoscope to Lachlan and took out a tiny bag mask unit to put over the baby's mouth and nose and provide the first breaths.

The disc of the stethoscope looked huge against the baby's chest but it was moving as air filled the small lungs and when Lachlan's gaze caught Pippa's she found she could breathe again as well.

'Heart rate's over a hundred,' he said. 'And look…he's pinking up.'

The baby took a breath for himself as Pippa lifted the mask and he was beginning to move his arms and legs. As the paediatric team rushed into the room, he began a wobbly cry that gained strength with his next breath. Pippa stepped back to let the paediatric consultant take over but she was smiling as she turned back to Ashley.

'Can you hear that?' she asked. 'That's your baby boy. He's doing well…'

She caught Lachlan's gaze again as she was turning.

His look was telling her that *they* had done well, too.

There was nobody else in the staffroom this soon after the shift change that day.

Just Pippa, who needed a moment to wind down before she got on with the rest of her day. She was sitting at the table, half a mug of coffee in front of her, just staring into space.

No wonder Lachlan looked surprised when he walked in and saw her.

'You still here? I would have thought you'd be hanging out to get home after a day like today.'

'I went to NICU to check on Ashley's baby.'

'Ah…how is he? I got caught up in Theatre after that excitement.'

'He's good. They're going to monitor him overnight, just to be on the safe side, but there's no indication of any neurological damage. Ashley would love a chance to thank you if you're going past the unit.'

'I'll make a point of doing that.' But Lachlan pulled out a chair and sat down opposite Pippa. 'As soon as I've sat down for two minutes. It's been quite a day.'

'It has.'

'I'm glad I've got the chance to tell you what a great job you did. I was…impressed.'

She ducked her head a little shyly at the praise. But then she risked an upward glance.

'So was I,' she said softly.

'It's not the first time I've thought that we make a good team,' Lachlan said. 'Maybe we should celebrate that with another prosecco at the pub one of these days.'

Pippa gave him another one of those stern looks—like she had when they'd been having that first prosecco.

Lachlan looked over his shoulder as if he wanted to make sure they were still alone. They were, but he lowered his voice anyway.

'You did get a chance to check that rule book of yours, I presume?'

'Um…yes.' Pippa bit her lip. This wasn't the first time she'd regretted making that throwaway comment.

'And was it in the section for professional relationships or the one that deals with dating? No… let me guess. It was in both, right?'

Pippa nodded.

'I like dating rules.' Lachlan's tone was approving. 'I have a few of my own.'

'Like what?'

'Like keeping things *strictly* casual. That's non-negotiable.'

'A "friends with benefits" kind of rule?'

'Exactly. But there's a time limit as well. And that removes any possibility that someone will expect commitment.'

'Sounds like a version of the "three date" rule.'

Lachlan made a sound that suggested he was intrigued. 'I think I've heard about that one somewhere.' He grinned. 'Probably in a dentist's waiting room magazine, but I didn't get time to read it properly. Do you use it? Is it as useful as the prosecco rule? What was the verdict on that one, anyway?'

Oh, help...

Pippa had dug herself a rather deep hole here, hadn't she?

Why on earth had she thrown in that stupid line about a 'three date' rule?

She knew why. It was automatic to pull any available cloak of protection around herself. Lachlan only had to talk to someone like Rita and he could find out she was single. Maybe she wanted to let him think that was by choice and not simply because she didn't have the courage to go anywhere near a relationship of any significance. How embarrassing would it be to admit she hadn't been in any kind of relationship, in fact, since her marriage had ended several years ago?

At least the question she needed to answer was on a different, imaginary, rule about going to a pub with your boss.

She caught his gaze again, fully intending to tell him that going out with the boss was definitely not permissible but...dammit...that eye contact unleashed one of those explosions of sparks. The man's attractiveness made him a kind of walking, talking firework, didn't it?

Pippa found herself shrugging. And saying something completely different.

'It could be up for negotiation.' She tried to sound as if success was unlikely. 'If the proper application forms are filled in.'

Lachlan nodded approvingly. 'Forms are good,' he said. 'Now...tell me how the "three date" rule works.'

She'd read about it herself. Quite possibly in a magazine.

'It does what it says on the tin,' she said. 'You get three dates and that's it. Both parties know the rules in advance, so it keeps things casual and makes it easy to back off but stay friends, if that's what either party wants.'

'Sounds perfect,' Lachan said thoughtfully. 'So...what about the subclauses?'

'Like what?'

'What constitutes a date? And...is sex on the agenda? On the first date even, given that the time limit's going to be rather restricted. I mean, this is kind of like a "friends with benefits" but with a use-by date, yes?'

Oh-h... Pippa couldn't respond to the query. He'd said the 's' word and her brain had turned to absolute mush. She was staring at Lachlan's hands, for heaven's sake. Imagining what it would be like to have his fingers trailing over her skin. It felt as if it could be dangerous. They might leave a flicker of tiny flames in their wake...

She cleared her throat. 'A date is any private meeting or shared activity that's agreed on in advance and...um...yes, it goes further than the boundaries of friendship, so it probably includes some form of...um...physical interaction.'

'Ah...so...if you happen to meet at a supermarket and end up in the pub drinking prosecco, it doesn't count?'

'No...' Pippa's tone was very firm. 'That was definitely not a *date*, Mr Smythe. If it's something that any friends can do, it doesn't count.'

He was smiling again. 'Clearly, I have a lot to learn,' he said. 'And from past experience I've found that the best way to learn something new is to give it a go. To get hands on.' His smile widened. 'So to speak...'

Pippa shook her head. 'Go for it,' she said. 'Did you have someone in mind to try it out on?'

Lachlan was looking up at the ceiling now, as if deep in thought. 'Absolutely,' he said a moment later. 'There is a contender.'

Pippa was, she had to admit, decidedly envious. She was also dead curious, but she managed to keep her tone casual.

'Who would that be?'

Lachlan's gaze flicked back to capture hers. '*You*, of course. Who else?'

CHAPTER FIVE

LACHLAN HAD BEEN CORRECT.

This could well be *perfect*.

A time limit. Three opportunities to have time together that could be romantic. Physical. Pleasurable and unforgettable.

It was not only permission to indulge in the satisfaction of an unusually intense attraction, it also had the potential to end as amicably as it had begun.

He did need to confirm that it was a good idea, mind you. Or rather, to make sure that Pippa was genuinely on board for what could only ever be a friendship with temporary benefits. Just a bit of a fling to defuse an attraction that could otherwise become something of a distraction.

A workplace liaison wasn't ideal, of course, especially when he'd only just started in a new position, and particularly one in the department he was now the head of, but perhaps that was even more of a reason to get it out of the way. It was quite obvious that the physical pull was mutual. Lachlan had actually seen her pupils dilate when he'd asked whether a first date could include sex and the way she'd been so flustered and determined not to let the word cross her own lips had been...

...adorable.

But it was equally clear that she had her doubts, and that was understandable. It *was* a bit of a minefield. If it went wrong it could damage not only his reputation at Queen Mary's but the excellent working relationship he was building with one of his most senior midwives.

Which turned out to be exactly what was making Pippa hesitant when Lachlan finally got an unexpected chance to speak to her in a place that couldn't have been more private. And secure.

The drug storage room—with a door that locked itself automatically when it closed behind the person authorised to enter. Pippa came in as Lachlan was about to leave. He didn't even need to raise the topic as he took a step towards the door. His raised eyebrows and a smile were enough to reveal that she'd been thinking about it. As much as he had?

'No,' she said. 'We work together. We'll still have to work together after the three dates. And you're my *boss*.'

'We're part of the same team,' he corrected

her. 'I'm quite confident we're both professional enough not to let something personal interfere with our ability to do our jobs. Who knows?' He tried to amp up the charm in his smile. 'Getting to know each other better might *improve* our working relationship.'

'Can you countersign a drug for me, please? That way I won't have to wait for Sally.'

'Sure.'

Pippa used a code to unlock the cabinet where the controlled drugs like narcotics were kept. She took an ampoule of morphine from a box, recorded her action in the logbook and signed her name.

Lachlan scribbled his initials in the final column as witness to the drug and quantity that had been removed. Pippa locked the cabinet again, put the ampoule into a kidney dish and then glanced up, her eyes narrowing.

'How do I know you're going to stick to the rules?'

'I'm good at rules.' Lachlan let himself sound slightly offended. 'I have my own rules about things. Like marriage.' He held his hands up. 'Not that I've had the same degree of trauma that you've had, but I'm on board with your aversion to it—and, presumably, to any long-term relationship that resembles marriage. I think we're on exactly the same page. I need to learn about this "three date" rule. I think it might serve me very well for the rest of my life. I can travel whenever I like, not collect any unwelcome baggage and… I might make some very good friends along the way—including you. Is that enough to convince you?'

'Hmm…' Pippa was adding an alcohol wipe, syringe and a needle to the kidney dish. The way she had her lips pressed together was giving away the fact that she was trying not to smile. Or appear too eager to give in?

Oh, man… Lachlan was seriously tempted to kiss Pippa right now. They were quite safe in here because there was no window on the solid door to get into this secure space and anyone coming in, like Sally was about to, would have to pause to use their swipe card. But that would hardly be the way to confirm that he was capable of behaving in a completely professional manner, was it? It was bad enough that he'd followed her into a locked room.

Not that she was making his restraint any easier. There was a glint in her eyes that told him she knew exactly what he was thinking and that she was not averse to the idea of being kissed. Something had to be done before this got out of hand, Lachlan decided. He was going to invite her to a first date. If her response made him feel like he was pushing her into something she was dubious about, he would back off and dismiss the prospect of even a single date with Pippa, let alone three of them.

'Let's do dinner,' he suggested. 'At the White Swan. I don't know if you noticed their blackboard menu, but they do steak and chips.'

Pippa lost the battle not to smile. 'I think you'll find that all pubs do steak and chips.'

'With an *egg*?'

She laughed. 'Maybe not always with an egg. Sometimes it can be with mushrooms.' She picked up the kidney dish. 'Excuse me, I've got someone who's pretty keen to get some more effective pain relief on board now that it's been charted.'

Lachlan stood between Pippa and the door for just a heartbeat longer. 'Is that a yes?'

'Will you stop waiting for me in locked rooms if I say yes?'

'Absolutely. Consider it a new rule.' He held the door open for Pippa.

She avoided making eye contact as she went past, and if anyone had been in the corridor outside they wouldn't have had any idea that her comment was about anything personal.

'Wednesday's probably good for me. Or Thursday. Let me know when you've checked your roster.'

* * *

Thursday.

Seven forty-five p.m.

Pippa was waiting, as arranged, by the bus stop near the staff parking area of the hospital—maybe a ten-minute walk away from the White Swan. Where she was about to go.

On a date.

With Lachlan Smythe.

Was it a date? She'd already been there with him, and that had definitely *not* been a date. But since then, that sizzling attraction had gone up by several noticeable notches. And he'd told her that he wanted to experience that imaginary 'three date' rule she had pretended to live by. It seemed that he was going to play by her rules and she had said that it was only a 'date' if there was some kind of physical interaction that wouldn't be appropriate if they were only friends.

A kiss.

More than a kiss.

A lot more than a kiss?

Good grief. Pippa was suddenly starting to feel all hot and bothered. Maybe this wasn't such a good idea, after all. But it was too late to back out now. She could see Lachlan striding towards her.

His smile was enough to make any doubts about what she was doing evaporate.

Dear Lord…the man was irresistible. Pippa decided she wasn't going to even think about any potentially negative consequences to this…date. Yep. She couldn't deny that she was hoping for an evening that would include some very inappropriate physical interaction.

'Hungry?' Lachlan asked.

'Starving.' Pippa nodded.

'Me, too.'

The words were a low, sexy growl. Pippa considered but then rejected making the suggestion that they skipped the pub and went straight to her place. She actually was very hungry. And this… anticipation was as delicious as any meal was going to be. Why not let it last a little longer?

The route to the White Swan meant they needed to cross one of the busy main roads that went through Richmond and had some residential houses with parking bays in front of them on one side and business premises on the other. Traffic was heading towards them from a distance as they crossed two lanes of the road to the central raised traffic island in front of an enormous supermarket delivery lorry and then waited for the bus that was coming in the opposite direction.

The blaring of an airhorn from the lorry was too close for comfort and they turned to see a car that was backing swiftly out from a parking space in front of a row of terraced houses, straight into the path of the truck. The driver swerved to miss the collision but was struggling for control as the huge vehicle rocked and it was already on the wrong side of the road. They could actually see the horror on the face of the bus driver as he realised what was happening. He was wrenching his steering wheel and the bus began heading straight for a big tree on the side of the road. The lorry hit the back of the bus with a sickening crunch at the same time the driver's end scraped past the tree with a screech of ripping metal and came to a shuddering halt. The impact was hard enough to shake the concrete island that Pippa and Lachlan were standing on.

There was noise everywhere now. Squealing from brakes being slammed on and crunching sounds from nose to tail collisions. There were horns blaring and people shouting. A faint scream was coming from inside the bus. A siren started as a police car in the distance raced to get to the scene. The thing that Pippa was most aware of in those first seconds, however, was that Lachlan's immediate reaction had been to grab hold of her.

To *protect* her.

And his first words, as he shielded her with his body, were to ask if she was okay.

'I'm fine,' she assured him. 'Oh, my God, Lachlan. We need to *do* something. Where do we start?'

'Triage,' he said. 'There'll be paramedics here in a matter of minutes but we can do a first sweep and at least make sure an airway is open if they're unconscious and get pressure on any uncontrolled bleeding.'

The lorry driver was climbing down from his cab that had jack-knifed after clipping the bus. He had blood streaming from a wound on his forehead. People were coming out of nearby shops, gathering to watch in horror. An elderly man on the other side of the road was standing beside the car that had caused the accident and drivers and passengers were getting out of their cars as they found themselves in a traffic snarl. A police officer was shouting at them to get back into their vehicles and move on so that the emergency services could get through.

'Come with me,' Lachlan directed.

The bus driver had managed to open the doors and he was leaning out.

'Help…we need *help*…'

Lachlan walked swiftly past the gathering crowd. 'There could be uninjured people coming out of the bus soon,' he told them. 'Keep them here and look after them until an ambulance arrives and they can be cleared.'

Pippa followed Lachlan into the bus through the back door. Shocked-looking people were sitting, immobile, still clinging onto the bars of the seats as if the bus was still moving. One man was standing in the aisle towards the back of the bus, bent over with his arms around his chest, and he was groaning loudly.

'If you can move, please make your way to the front of the bus,' Lachlan called loudly. 'There are people outside who will help you.'

The worst of the damage was at the back of the bus, where the side had been caved in and the windows shattered. A crumpled figure was lying across the back seat. A window on the other side had also been broken by a branch of the tree that was now inside the bus and someone was hunched inside the greenery, their hands covering their head.

People further up the bus were beginning to stand up and move cautiously towards the front door.

'Can you check the guy in the tree?' Lachlan asked. 'And have a look for anyone that might have slipped down between the seats as well. I need to get to that person on the back seat.'

But he paused as he went past the man holding his chest. 'Are you having trouble breathing?'

'It hurts…' The man groaned again. 'I was

waiting to get off at the next stop and… I hit my ribs on the pole.'

Pippa could see Lachlan helping the man to sit down carefully on the nearest seat before he moved swiftly past. She had reached the man half-hidden amongst the foliage of the tree. She could see blood trickling through his fingers.

'Can you hear me?' she asked.

'Y-yes…'

'Did the branch hit you? Were you knocked out?'

'I…don't think so. But… I'm bleeding.'

'I can see that.' Pippa was breaking off the leafy twigs to clear a space. It looked as though this man had been incredibly lucky and the larger branches had only skimmed his head enough to give him the kind of scalp laceration that was notorious for bleeding heavily. 'Is it hard to breathe at all?'

'No…'

'Anything else hurting?'

'No…'

'Okay… Don't move. I'll be back soon, but there will be more help arriving any second.'

A lot of the passengers had managed to get off the bus now, with the help of the driver and people outside. By the time Pippa had checked the floor between the seats and turned back, she could see the flashing lights of both fire service and ambulance vehicles arriving. She could also see Lachlan perched on the back seat, his hands positioned to keep the airway of an unconscious person open. As she tried to get back to check on the man with the scalp wound, paramedics were coming in through both doors of the bus. One team went straight to Lachlan. Another to the man who was holding his ribs.

'Are you hurt?'

Pippa turned to the paramedic who'd come in through the front door.

'You're covered in blood,' they added.

'Am I?' Pippa glanced down and found that her pale green shirt was, indeed, streaked with blood. She shook her head. 'I'm fine… I'm a nurse. First on the scene with a doctor.' This blood must have come from the leafy twigs she'd been breaking and moving. 'There's someone with a scalp laceration beside that tree branch.'

'Right.' They were already moving. 'Thanks for your help. We've got this now.'

Pippa climbed off the bus. Someone jumped out of the back of an ambulance and, having heard her story, gave her a pump bottle of hand sanitiser and a towel to clean any blood off her hands.

'Are you vaccinated for hepatitis?'

'Yes.'

The paramedic was peering at her face. 'You

should be okay. Can't see any splashes around your eyes or mouth. I'm guessing you're well aware of protocols for contact with blood or body fluids.'

'I'll be fine.' But Pippa had a moment of concern for Lachlan. What was he still doing in the bus? Was he putting himself at more risk than she had? She stood to one side of the scene, waiting for him to appear, watching firemen and more ambulance officers entering the bus with equipment, including a rescue basket. A short time later, the most seriously injured passenger was brought out, strapped into the basket stretcher. He was in a cervical collar and had an oxygen mask covering his face. Lachlan was walking behind the stretcher and followed it to the ambulance, where it was loaded, the vehicle moving off seconds later with its lights flashing.

Pippa watched Lachlan turn to scan the scene as the ambulance left. That he was looking for her was obvious by the way his face relaxed when he spotted her. As he walked towards her, Pippa was aware of a curious melting sensation deep inside her body. She was remembering the way he hadn't hesitated to shield her as soon as he'd realised something dangerous was happening around them. How long had it been since anyone had cared for her like that?

Too long…

Lachlan noticed the blood smears on her shirt as quickly as the paramedic had.

'Not mine,' she assured him.

'I'm probably a mess myself,' he said. 'I certainly feel like I could use a hot shower and a change of clothes.' He took another glance around them. 'We're don't need to be here any longer but... I don't think we're going to get anywhere near the White Swan tonight.'

'No...we might need a rain check on that.' Pippa checked her watch. 'Good grief...it's after nine p.m. I had no idea we'd been here this long.'

'That guy in the back seat needed a bit of work. He regained consciousness but had enough of a head injury to be combative and need sedation.' He blew out a breath. 'Let me walk you home, at least.'

She shook her head. 'You'd be even further away from that shower and the clean clothes. I'll be home in a few minutes. It's all good.'

'If you're sure.' But Lachlan was hesitating. He made a rueful face. 'Not much of a first date, was it?'

'It doesn't count,' Pippa said. 'And, even it if did, it certainly wasn't boring.'

Lachlan was smiling again. 'It wasn't, was it? So I get another shot at a first date?'

Pippa could still feel the warmth of that being cared for feeling. She smiled back at him.

'It would be a bit rude to say no, wouldn't it?'

'Absolutely. 'Night, Pippa.' Lachlan dipped his head and brushed her cheek with his lips. 'We'll have better luck next time.'

Again, she was watching him. His back, this time, as he headed in the direction they'd come from. He lifted his hand in another gesture of farewell and Pippa lifted her own, even though she knew he couldn't see it. Then she found herself touching her cheek.

It hadn't been a real kiss but she could still feel its imprint.

She wished it *had* been real.

Both the date and the kiss.

CHAPTER SIX

THE FRUSTRATION WAS REAL.

The closest Lachlan got to seeing Pippa in the next couple of days was a photograph that appeared in the local newspaper, of the accident scene on the night of what was supposed to have been their first date, taken when she was getting out of the bus with all those blood stains on her shirt.

He hadn't forgotten the feeling of wondering whether she'd been injured herself, clambering around inside that bus. Or that overwhelming urge to keep her safe when he'd seen the dreadful accident unfolding in front of their eyes—so close it felt as if they'd escaped death themselves.

Was fate trying to warn him to stay away from her?

Was that why it was proving so difficult to catch even a moment with her during work hours, so they could at least find a time to try again?

It wasn't going to happen today, that was certain. Lachlan had checked the roster this morning—something that was perfectly legitimate for him to do, given that he was the HoD—and found that Pippa was on the first of two days off.

He'd worked late, being on call and having had an emergency Caesarean that he'd only just finished. He wasn't covering the night shift but the surgery had started just before the change-over and it had been a complicated and time-consuming case because the mother had dense adhesions from previous C-sections. She had lost a lot of blood and was being kept overnight in the ICU for monitoring due to a dip in the level of her kidney function. Lachlan wanted to check on her again before he went home for the night. By the time he was satisfied that she was doing well, it was nearly midnight and he was more than ready to go home.

Until he was on the way to the car park, when he spotted Pippa outside the hospital, sitting on a bench beside an archway that invited people to enter the garden area that was a feature of The Queen Mary Hospital's grounds. She was wearing scrubs and had a packet of sandwiches on her lap that looked as if they'd been spat out of a hospital vending machine.

'Pippa! What on earth are you doing here at this time of night? It's your day off, isn't it?'

'How did you know that?'

'Ah…' Should he look embarrassed that he'd been stalking her? The way she'd been when she'd paid attention to what was being said on the hospital grapevine. No… He sat down beside her instead. 'It doesn't matter,' he said. 'It's good to see you.'

'I'm not supposed to be here,' Pippa admitted. 'I came in last minute because they were so short-staffed, and I've got tomorrow off so I can catch up on sleep. They're being kind to me. They said to take as long as I like for a dinner break and they'll only page me if I'm really needed.'

'Excellent. That'll give us time to arrange another date. Oh, wait…it wasn't a date last time, was it?'

'No…' Pippa looked down at the sandwiches she was holding. Lachlan could see that their corners were curled up and there was a tired-looking lettuce leaf poking out. 'Steak and chips sound pretty good right now.'

'I think I can do better than that,' Lachlan said. 'I think we deserve more than a pub dinner after the disaster the other night. What's the best restaurant in Richmond?'

'What's your favourite food?'

'Italian.'

'There are some amazing Italian restaurants in Richmond.'

'But what's *your* favourite food?' Lachlan hadn't forgotten the meal ingredients he'd seen in her supermarket trolley. 'When you go out, that is?'

'Probably French.'

'Is there an amazing French restaurant in Richmond?'

'There is.' Pippa was smiling, as if she was pleased with the direction this conversation was going in. '*Chez Anton*. It's right by the river and I've never been.' She hesitated, as if she was wondering whether to explain why that might be. 'It's a bit posh,' she added.

'Then that's where we'll go,' Lachlan said. 'Tomorrow night, seven p.m.'

'Okay... I can meet you there. It's an easy walk for me.' Pippa's eyes were shining and her lips were parted and...

...and she looked totally irresistible.

Lachlan couldn't look away from her eyes and it seemed as if Pippa wasn't about to break that eye contact, even when he leaned close enough to make it more than apparent that he was thinking of kissing her.

If anything, it felt as if she was leaning towards *him*.

It didn't matter. The important thing was that their lips were touching and...oh, man...it was just as delicious as he'd known it would be. He moved his lips over hers and could feel her response as a tiny gasp as he touched her bottom lip with his tongue. The pressure of the kiss changed and there was an urgent note to it now. They both wanted more…

Perhaps it was just as well that Pippa's pager sounded at the precise moment things were tipping into something far too intense, given that they were sitting where anybody coming out of Queen Mary's might see them. Lachlan might not know all the rules in Pippa's book but he could be fairly sure there could very well be something about keeping it private and protecting reputations.

That didn't magically erase the frustration, but it helped considerably that Pippa was feeling it, too. Lachlan felt her sigh against his lips as she broke the contact.

'I have to go,' she whispered.

'I know.' Lachlan found a smile as he remembered something that really did help deal with that unresolved tension. 'See you tomorrow night, Pippa.'

She couldn't stop thinking about it.

That *kiss*…

Every time she thought about it, her entire body felt as if it was melting. Especially when she finally climbed into her bed the next morning to get a few hours' sleep. Even more so in the evening as she got ready to go out.

On a date that was very likely to include another kiss.

Pippa had never felt quite this nervous about a date. Or taken quite so much care to look her absolute best. When her freshly washed hair was dry, she used her straighteners to turn it into a shiny fall that felt like silk rippling on her bare shoulders, because it was still warm enough on this summer's evening to wear a sundress that had spaghetti straps that were tied in bows, a shirred bodice and a long skirt that was full enough to swirl around her legs. It was her favourite colour, a soft olive green, with a print of tiny white daisies, and she kept her accessories simple, with leather sandals on her feet and thin silver bangles on her wrist. The walk along the towpath beside the river was one she loved but she barely noticed the boats or dog walkers or the band setting up to play live music in one of the restaurant gardens this evening.

All she could think about was Lachlan Smythe.

And that *kiss*.

He was waiting for her outside *Chez Anton* and he was looking as summery as Pippa, in a cream open-necked, short-sleeved shirt and sand-coloured chinos. They were shown to a table in the garden, shaded by a lush grapevine, that overlooked a grassy bank, the towpath and a wide stretch of the river and the waiter handed them menus.

'Can I get you something to drink?'

Pippa caught Lachlan's gaze. She wanted to ask for a glass of prosecco, but she had to make it seem as if she was following known rules for a casual relationship and having a drink that linked them as a couple had to be a no-no.

'I can recommend the house champagne,' the waiter said.

'Sounds perfect,' Lachlan said.

'Yes, please,' Pippa said.

Lachlan waited until the waiter walked away to wink at Pippa. 'Champagne is just the French version of prosecco,' he murmured. He opened his menu. 'And look…they do steak and chips.'

'It'll be *steak frites* here. No eggs.'

'Doesn't béarnaise sauce have egg in it?'

Pippa had to laugh. 'I do believe it does. Egg yolks, anyway.'

But there it was. Another connection. Was that why it felt as if there was a genuine friendship between them already? And was *that* what was making this attraction something unlike anything Pippa had ever felt, even with the man she had fallen in love with enough and ended up marrying?

They drank the champagne and ate the crispiest twice-cooked French fries with slivers of steak that were tender enough to melt in their mouths and deliciously coated with the tarragon and chervil flecked sauce. They had crème brûlée for dessert, along with another glass of champagne, and they still hadn't run out of things to talk about. The conversation had, in fact, naturally become more personal.

'I couldn't stay in Birmingham after my marriage ended,' Pippa told him. 'And it was the best thing I ever did to move here. I absolutely love being so close to the river. I walk along here on the towpath every chance I get.'

'Do you cycle?'

'I used to, when I was a kid.'

'I passed a place where you can hire bicycles. Think how far you could go on the Thames Path on a bike.'

'How far would you want to go?'

'Pangbourne Meadows.'

'What? Why?'

'It's supposed to be one of the best places for wild swimming near London.'

'Oh?' Pippa focused on scraping up the last morsel of her dessert. She wasn't going to let herself think about that snippet of gossip where the suggestion had been made that the new HoD might go swimming naked.

'Petersham Meadows is also good, apparently,' Lachlan continued. 'And that's probably walking distance from here.'

'Mmm…' Pippa was thinking of somewhere that was even more within walking distance.

Her cottage.

Her bedroom.

Suddenly aware of an unusual silence, she looked up to find Lachlan's gaze resting on her.

'Shall we head off?' he asked softly.

There was a new tension between them as they walked away from the restaurant.

Who was going to say something first? Or would nothing be said and they would get back to wherever Lachlan had parked his car and then they'd say goodnight and that would be the end of the date?

Pippa didn't want it to be the end.

The band that had been setting up as Pippa had been walking in the other direction was still playing as they went past. The lead singer was a woman with an amazing voice and they stopped to listen to her rendition of Prince's 'Nothing Compares 2 U'.

They were standing so close together that their arms were touching and it felt as natural as breathing to link their hands. And then Lachlan slipped his hand around her waist and… they were dancing. Just swaying together to start with, but then Lachlan lifted his arm and Pippa turned beneath it, stepping further away to let Lachlan pull her back, even more closely, into his arms. And then she rested her head in the hollow beneath his shoulder and he rested his cheek on her hair. When the song ended, they looked at each other and it turned out that there was very little that needed to be said.

Only four words, in fact, and it was Lachlan who whispered them.

'Your place or mine?'

Pippa's place.

The tiniest, cutest cottage Lachlan had ever seen, with its pink door between two square windows and a wisteria vine that had tendrils long enough to catch in his hair as he followed Pippa inside.

It could have been a garden shed for all he cared, mind you. He just wanted to be behind a closed door, in a space where he could be completely alone with Pippa. It felt as if he'd been waiting for this moment for…for ever?

He was holding her hand as they went inside. By tacit consent, they both stood there in silence, very still, as their eyes got accustomed to the reduced level of light. Until they could see each other just as well as they needed to.

Lachlan could see the shine of Pippa's hair

and he wove his fingers into the thickness of it behind her head and let it ripple through them like silky ribbons. She closed her eyes as if she could feel it as well. Her lips parted and…

…and Lachlan was lost.

He touched his lips to hers. So softly it was no more than a breath. And then again, catching her lower lip between his and touching it with his tongue. A tiny sound came from Pippa—just a catch of her breath, but it was enough for him to cover her mouth again, and this time it was a real kiss. A conversation of pressure and response, lips and tongues, hands that were moving on bare skin and desire that was spiralling into a level that Lachlan had never known existed. Even if he had, he might well have avoided going anywhere near it, because it was redolent of a lack of control that was both unacceptable and intoxicatingly compelling.

Those stringy straps of Pippa's dress had bows and all it needed was a tug to undo them. He lifted his head enough to catch her gaze as he untied them because he needed to be sure that she wanted this as much as he did, but she was looking down, her fingers starting to unbutton his shirt. Maybe she felt the urgency in his gaze because her fingers stilled and, a beat later, she lifted her chin and met his gaze.

He could see the heat of desire in her eyes and

there was no doubt that she wanted this to continue. There was a kind of wonder there as well, as though she didn't quite believe the power of what was happening between them and…oh, Lord…was that a hint of fear in there, too?

He hadn't expected that from someone who made her own rules and then followed them to the letter. He hadn't expected the…vulnerability he could see and that touched something that was deeper than purely physical.

He held her gaze and what he said came straight from his heart.

'You're safe,' he said softly. 'You can trust me.'

'I know…' She was the one holding *his* gaze now and the edges of any fear had softened. 'You can trust me, too.'

Her bedroom was on the other side of the narrow hallway down the centre of the cottage and there wasn't much space to walk around her bed, which was fine as far as Lachlan was concerned. The bed was the only space they needed. The rest of the world was about to become completely irrelevant.

They stood at the end of the bed to undress each other. He heard Pippa's gasp when his hands brushed her breasts as he pulled down the stretchy top of her dress. It was his turn to make a sound like a groan when she was undoing the leather belt of his chinos.

'Wait…' He reached into his pocket to find the foil packet that was inside his wallet.

'You don't have to,' Pippa whispered. 'I'm on the Pill.'

Lachlan leaned in to kiss her. 'Consider it an insurance policy,' he murmured. 'You can never be too careful.'

He never had—and never *would*—let anyone else take the responsibility for something this important.

Once he knew he was safe, that they were both safe, then he could let himself sink into what was promising to be the best sex he'd ever experienced. Ever…

Oh, *my*…

That was about as coherent as Pippa's thoughts were for quite some time.

It wasn't just the way Lachlan was touching her, with his hands and his tongue, his soft words and the sounds of pleasure—ecstasy, even—that he made. It was the feel of *his* skin beneath her hands and the taste of him and…the way they could move together that made it feel impossible that this was the first time.

It wasn't until she was lying there, waiting

for her pulse and breathing to get a lot closer to normal, that reality began to take shape again.

Maybe it was the sound of Lachlan's breath that was halfway to being a sigh.

'Strike one,' he said.

Pippa blinked. 'What?'

'I'm guessing this counts as a date.' There was an amused note in his voice now.

'Oh…' Pippa turned her head. Her nose was almost touching Lachlan's. 'Yes,' she added. 'Definitely a date.'

'So that's number one.'

'It is.' Pippa tried to sound solemn but it was difficult when she was feeling this *good*. And happy. Lachlan wanting to experiment with the 'three date' rule meant that it could happen again.

Twice, in fact.

Lachlan was clearly following the same thought process. He kissed Pippa softly.

'Only two left,' he said.

Pippa nodded. But she caught her bottom lip between her teeth to stop herself smiling. Thank goodness she hadn't come up with the notion of a 'one date' rule.

'Okay if I have a shower before I head home?'

'Of course.'

Lachlan swung his legs over the side of the

bed, but then he seemed to freeze. For long enough for Pippa to feel herself frowning.

'You okay?'

'I'm...not sure...'

Pippa propped herself up on her elbow. 'Why?'

'Ah...the condom broke.' His words were a monotone. 'That's never happened to me before.'

'It's okay,' Pippa said. 'Like I said, I'm on the Pill. And I haven't missed any doses recently. I've had years of practice.'

The glance over his shoulder was surprised enough to make Pippa blush.

'Not because I have an overactive sex life. And I've never had an STI so you're also safe on that count. You're actually the first in quite a while.' Pippa pulled the duvet up to cover herself. 'I used to get irregular cycles, that's all. And menorrhagia. Enough to get anaemic.'

Lachlan was nodding. 'You're safe, too,' he said. 'So...' He got to his feet. 'All good, then.'

Pippa watched him walk to her tiny bathroom. Tall, lean and totally naked.

Yeah...it was definitely all good.

About as good as anything could ever get.

CHAPTER SEVEN

IT WAS ALL very well having another two dates to look forward to, but it would be way too easy to use them up in as many days, wouldn't it?

Lachlan saw Pippa at the central desk as he walked past, the morning after date number one, and he could feel the burning embers from the night before as clearly as if he were walking over hot coals. It was extremely tempting to get to his office as quickly as possible and fire off a text message to find out if she might be free this evening for dinner or a show or something.

Especially the something.

Even the most fleeting flashback to the finale of last night's date was enough to cause flames to reignite from those embers and ramp up the heat. The kind of heat that should trigger a smoke alarm in the ward, let alone any internal warning system, but Lachlan was comfortable that this was safe.

For whatever reason—and he suspected it had a lot to do with the failure of her marriage—

Pippa had strict rules about dating that she was currently following in her personal life.

Lachlan's were even stricter. He didn't know if he carried the Huntington gene himself. He'd never been tested and he didn't want to be. Having had years to think about it before he'd turned eighteen and could choose for himself, he'd decided it was preferable to live his life without knowing that the Sword of Damocles was hanging over his head. If he started to show symptoms, he'd deal with it then. What he would never do, however, was to let someone else get close enough for them to be affected as well because that would be as bad as passing the gene onto an innocent child. Almost...

He wasn't about to break the rules and try and extend the number of dates, no matter how much he might be tempted to, but even if he found the temptation irresistible he had the insurance policy that Pippa wouldn't be having a bar of it. This was a private and temporary arrangement and she was being very careful that their colleagues weren't going to suspect there was anything more than a professional relationship between them.

'Good morning, Mr Smythe.'

She wasn't giving the slightest hint of just how well they knew each other now. No wonder he was feeling so safe.

'Morning, Pippa.' Lachlan nodded at the staff members gathering for the handover. 'Rita… Sally—how are you?'

'I'm very good.' Sally grinned. 'Or so I've been led to believe.'

Lachlan gave a huff of laughter and kept moving, without looking back at Pippa.

Playing the game of keeping the 'three date' thing a secret might be as enjoyable as fighting the flames of desire every time they were close enough to be breathing the same air. It could add considerably to the anticipation of date two, in fact. How much hotter could things get, he wondered, if they kept each other waiting a bit?

A lot hotter, he decided when he managed to get to the cafeteria for a lunch break. Pippa was going in the other direction. He glanced at the plastic triangle sandwich pack in her hands and then lifted his gaze. It only took a heartbeat of eye contact to know they were both remembering the other night, when the first real date had been agreed on and Pippa had been holding exactly the same food. The subtle quirk of her eyebrow told him that, yeah…steak and chips might still be a preferable meal choice.

It felt like a private invitation to arrange another date.

The way her lips were curving into the merest suggestion of a smile as they carried on in opposite directions without even speaking to each other told him that his own expression had conveyed his intended message.

Soon. But not yet...

Who was going to broach the subject of a second date?

When several days had gone by without Lachlan saying anything, Pippa might have started wondering if he had decided that he didn't *want* a second date.

But she knew that wasn't true.

She could feel the hum in the air between them and she knew perfectly well that he could feel it as well. Fortunately, it was a hum that was quite controllable. It was automatically there as soon as they were anywhere near each other, but it came with a mental switch. It could be dimmed enough to be kept private, like when they were attending a staff meeting or they happened to be collecting sets of notes from the reception desk in Outpatients at the same time. It could be switched off completely when any personal interaction was totally inappropriate, which was any instance of them both being involved in a birth that required some medical intervention.

Or was it more that the personal hum was overridden by a professional one when that happened?

Because it did feel different to be working with Lachlan than with other consultants. Just having him in the room for the end of the second stage of a breech delivery, a week after their date, was enough to keep the atmosphere calm, even when it became apparent that a serious complication could be developing.

'You're doing really well, Amber. Baby's legs and bottom are born now. Take a few deep breaths and then have a wiggle and start pushing again.'

But Pippa was watching the baby's body carefully and there was no sign of the expected rotation that would put the back uppermost. She glanced up at the clock. The minutes were ticking past and it was a short window. There should be a steady descent of the baby's head and it should appear within three minutes of the umbilicus being born. Amber was pushing again but there was still no progress.

Pippa knew the three-minute mark had passed as Lachlan stepped closer.

'I'm just going to check on what's happening,' he warned Amber. 'Don't push. Take a few more breaths.'

The episiotomy Pippa had performed made it easier for Lachlan to slip his hand in as gently as possible. She saw his expression change moments later.

'Bilateral extended arms,' he said quietly.

The baby's head was stuck because of the extra room needed with the arms on either side. Pippa knew Lachlan would be trying to flex the baby's elbow and sweep an arm out. She also knew you only made one attempt.

And it hadn't been successful.

'What's happening?' Amber's husband was helping her to breathe in the Entonox. He was looking very pale. 'Why isn't the baby moving?'

'He's got his arms up,' Pippa said. 'Which is making things a bit tight. He needs some help to get going again.'

Lachlan was holding the baby's pelvis now, with his forefingers on the back and his thumbs around the legs. Pippa watched him perform a procedure he was clearly very familiar with, lifting the baby's body and rotating it in one direction and then back again. The manoeuvre was designed to unlock the impaction and bring the arms in front of the body.

Pippa held her breath. She could see in Lachlan's face the moment he felt the movement of the baby and then she could see the arms and shoulders being born. He adjusted his hold, cradling the tiny body on one hand and putting his fingers on the back of the baby's head.

He glanced up.

'Suprapubic pressure?' Pippa was already getting her hand in position on Amber's belly.

'Thanks.'

Pippa pressed down firmly as Lachlan corrected the flexion that was making the head difficult to deliver and, finally, the baby was born. She felt as if she was taking a first breath along with the infant and she could hear—and feel—the relieved breath that Lachlan expelled. In the blink of time before the baby's breath became a cry, she shared a glance with Lachlan and it felt like a smile. An emergency had been averted. Her trust in his skills had continued its climb and the feeling that they were, indeed, a good team became even stronger—a professional hum that was just as significant as a personal one, especially a personal one that had a distinct time limit of its own.

Okay…

Enough was enough.

It was well over a week since their night together and Lachlan wanted to lock in a second date. It didn't have to be in the next day or two but he wanted confirmation that it *was* going to happen.

He texted Pippa.

Do you like West End musicals? Fancy dinner and a show?

The response came back fast enough to suggest that Pippa had also had enough of waiting.

Sounds great. But not tonight—I've got an antenatal class to run. And I'm back on night shifts again next week.

No problem. I'll get tickets and let you know.

Lachlan checked Pippa's roster to see what date she was starting her week of night shifts and booked tickets for an evening where neither of them had work the next day.

Just in case they didn't get much sleep that night…

His registrar rang to let him know they were ready to start a ward round in the post-surgical ward but Lachlan took a brief detour on the way, to stop at the reception desk in the labour ward.

'I don't know anything about the antenatal classes we're running,' he said to Rita. 'Where are they? And who's in charge?'

'There's a training room attached to the physiotherapy gymnasium,' Rita said. 'It's all set up with lots of birthing balls and plastic pelvises and slightly weird-looking fake babies.' She smiled at him. 'You know…the usual stuff. It's a four-week course, on Tuesdays from seven to nine p.m., and it's for women from about thirty weeks pregnant. The midwives do the majority of the teaching and they have a roster for it.' She looked over her shoulder. 'It's Pippa tonight and it's a Session Three. From memory, that's about active birthing positions and breathing techniques. I've heard it can get quite physical. Maybe you should pop in and see it for yourself.'

It wasn't a bad idea. Lachlan had another viewing of the house near Marble Hill Park because he hadn't been able to forget those gorgeous views across Richmond Park from the upstairs bedrooms. The idea of a legitimate reason to spend time with Pippa at work when he wasn't in a professional role himself was quite intriguing.

Lachlan smiled at Rita. 'I might just do that.'

Lachlan had no trouble finding the training room in the physiotherapy department later that evening because he could hear the voices and laughter from some distance away. He let himself quietly into the room, where half a dozen pregnant women and their birthing partners were in various positions around the room.

Pippa was rubbing the back of a woman who was on all fours on a padded mat.

'Don't let your lower back sag,' he heard her

saying. 'Curl it up and then straighten it. Pelvic tilts are great just for relaxation at the end of a long day, but they're also going to be great during labour.'

A father-to-be who looked young enough to still be a teenager was bouncing across the other side of the room on a large birthing ball. Pippa looked up and then started moving. Her eyes widened in surprise when she noticed Lachlan at the door, but she was on a mission.

'I hope you're not going to let Scarlett do that when she's in labour, Kyle. What did I say about bouncing?'

Kyle looked sheepish. 'That it can jam the baby in a bad position.'

'Close enough.'

'He's an idiot.' The pregnant young woman walking towards them was glaring at Kyle. 'Honestly, I can't take him anywhere. I have no idea why I let him get me pregnant.'

'You love me, babe.' Kyle was grinning. 'You couldn't resist my charms. Look… I know what to do. Rotate your hips, go from side to side. Do figure eights. I'm onto it.'

'Fabulous.' Pippa smiled at him. She raised her voice to get the attention of the rest of the class. 'Let's use the last bit of tonight's class to practise some of the breathing techniques we talked about earlier. Try the deep, slow, calming breaths. Inhale quietly. You can be as vocal as you want on the exhalation.'

She threw a grin in Lachlan's direction as loud groaning broke out, the birthing partners apparently keen to participate, and held up her hand, fingers splayed, to signal that she should be finishing up in five minutes or so.

Lachlan was more than happy to wait. He watched Pippa going from couple to couple, encouraging them, praising them and answering any questions they had. She was confident, friendly and warm and the class attendees clearly loved her, judging by their comments as they left.

'You're the best, Pippa,' one of them said. 'I'm keeping my fingers crossed that you're on duty when I come in to do this for real.'

'I didn't want to come,' Kyle confessed on his way out. 'But it was kinda cool.'

'I'll make sure he behaves himself better next time,' Scarlett said.

Pippa was smiling as she watched the young couple walking out of the room holding hands.

And Lachlan was smiling as he watched Pippa.

She was still in her working uniform of scrubs, with ugly but comfortable plastic clogs on her feet. Her hair was tamed into the familiar long braid and she was wearing no jewellery and minimal, if any, make-up and…

…and she was still one of the most beautiful women Lachlan had ever met.

But the sensation squeezing his chest right now was very different to the physical attraction that he'd been aware of from the moment he'd first laid eyes on Pippa Gordon. Attraction like that was something chemical. Something that would, inevitably, fade.

He respected how good Pippa was at her job and he really *liked* her as a person and they were both things that were very likely to get stronger rather than fading. Could they end up being real friends once the physical attraction wore off?

Close enough to at least partly fill that empty space in his life where special people should be?

That space that could feel so damn lonely sometimes?

His smile widened as the last couple left and Pippa walked towards him.

'What on earth are you doing *here*?'

'I heard about the classes. I thought a good head of department should be up to speed with everything going on. Plus… I was in the area. I went back to see that house off Richmond Road again.'

'Did you decide to buy it?'

'I did.'

Because it had happened again when he'd looked at the view over Richmond Park. The memories of times with his brother and his family had been even more vivid this time and it felt as if they had the power to shine a different kind of light into that empty space in his life. To be able to feel that those memories of the happiest time of his life were worth hanging on to—celebrating, even—instead of avoiding them because of the sadness attached to them was…well…it was breaking new ground for Lachlan. He could see clearly that, despite the pain that came later, he would never have chosen for that part of his life not to exist. He was, in fact, very grateful for it. He was going to welcome other memories. He might even go looking for old photographs that he could frame or hang on a wall. Because he was going to *have* walls of his own in the very near future.

'I put an offer in on it,' he told Pippa. 'And it was accepted.'

'Wow… Congratulations. That's exciting.'

Pippa started rolling a birthing ball to one side of the room. Lachlan went to pick up another one.

'It's certainly something to celebrate,' he agreed. 'And the White Swan will be my local in a matter of weeks.'

'Might need more than a cheeky prosecco at the local to celebrate something that big.'

'Perhaps we can find some champagne when we go to that show next Wednesday. I've got the tickets.'

'Oh, lovely… What are we going to see?'

'Let me surprise you. I'm sure you'll love it.'

'I'm sure I will.'

The look in Pippa's eyes made Lachlan think she wasn't referring to the latest musical extravaganza being put on in the West End and the flush of pink in her cheeks as she turned away to fetch another ball was all the confirmation he needed.

Perhaps she was going to be counting off the days to their second date with just as much anticipation as he would be. Not that he was about to admit that. Keeping things casual was obviously a foundation rule for the 'three date' game.

How good was it that they were both playing a game that had such well-structured rules? Neither of them was going to let things get out of control and when it ended—as it was destined to do—there would be no hard feelings and they would be able to remain friends.

Pippa could very well become the best friend Lachlan had ever had. Close enough for him to, one day, be able to tell her why anything more than friendship was impossible?

In the meantime, he could look forward to their next date and, inevitably, how their evening was going to end.

Lachlan had no reason to think that sex with Pippa wouldn't be as good the second time as it had been on their first date.

What was totally unexpected was that it turned out to be so much *better*.

Different.

Slower.

So much more intense.

He lay awake for a long time after he'd put Pippa safely into a taxi to get home from his apartment after an amazingly enjoyable night with a show they'd both loved, a riverside dinner—with champagne, of course—ending up in *his* bed, possibly because neither of them wanted to take the time to get back to Pippa's cottage in a different suburb.

It had felt like more than just sex.

In hindsight, it felt as if it had been dangerously close to being more than a purely physical connection.

It felt like they had been making love.

And that was breaking the rules that Pippa didn't know about. He was letting himself get too close to someone. If Pippa felt like this as well, she was going to end up being hurt.

Not nearly as hurt as she would be, however, if they went any further down the track of falling in love with each other. Or, heaven forbid, if she had to go through what he'd had to when he'd watched the struggle both his brother and his father had had to endure. To end up totally broken, like his mother, and simply give up on life.

Lachlan might not be able to protect himself if the worst was going to happen but he could protect someone he cared about. Tonight, he'd realised just how much he was starting to care about Pippa and it was enough for him to know he had to let her escape before any real harm was done.

He had to find a way to stop playing this game, preferably in a way that wouldn't have any negative impact on the friendship they were building and the professional relationship they already had.

He didn't quite know how he was going to do that.

He just knew that it was game over for him.

There simply couldn't be a third date and that was that.

The dream was so real, it was like making love to Lachlan Smythe all over again.

Pippa could feel the stroke of his hands on her skin and the slide of his tongue. She could hear the murmur of his voice and the groan of his pleasure. She could even feel the building of that exquisite pleasure that was almost pain, knowing that it was about to morph into a kaleidoscope of sensation that was simply pure bliss.

But then, in that odd way dreams could edit out chunks of time, she was watching Lachlan walk towards a door.

Naked—like he had been when she'd watched him walking to the bathroom in her cottage that first night. Except that she knew he wasn't going to a bathroom. He was about to walk out of her house.

Out of her life.

And it felt as if he was taking her whole world with him.

She tried to call out.

Don't go... Please don't go... Don't leave me...

The effort she put into trying to make a sound was so great that Pippa woke herself up.

She lay there in her bed, her breath coming in gasps, her body shaking, still caught by fragments of the dream, that fear of losing Lachlan so strong she knew exactly what it was.

She was falling in love with him.

This wasn't supposed to happen. This was supposed to have been safe. She knew that Lachlan wasn't remotely interested in anything more than a casual relationship. He'd been even more interested in one that had a use-by date.

There was no denying that it *was* happening, however. To *her*.

In the space of two dates? How much worse could it get with a third date?

Good grief. Pippa deliberately pulled in a deeper breath to try and persuade her body—and mind—to shake off the fear.

It couldn't happen. Pippa couldn't go back into that space where you gave someone your heart and they stomped on it until it was completely broken.

The dream was a warning she couldn't ignore.

Damage control was required. Somehow, she had to find a way to make sure that third date didn't happen.

CHAPTER EIGHT

THANK GOODNESS IT was getting easier.

For the first week or so after that second date, Pippa could feel wisps of that dream messing with her head every time she saw Lachlan at work. The pull towards him was a kind of force field she was having to fight not to get sucked into. For a few days she even wondered whether it was too late.

Had she already fallen in love with him?

No, of course she hadn't. Even if it was possible to fall in love that fast, she had an insurance policy of the agreement that they were both on the same page as far as relationships that could be considered in any way serious. And falling in love was about as serious as they got, wasn't it?

The professional distance they had always kept during working hours helped a lot. Lachlan was friendly but appropriately distant with her, just the way he was with other colleagues like Rita and Sally and Peter and it was just the reminder Pippa needed that falling for a man like Lachlan was guaranteed to break your heart. Had dating him at all been a mistake? Why was it that men seemed to be generally better than women at being able to have a completely casual relationship that included sex or a bit of fun like a 'three date' game without emotions getting in the way?

No. Pippa couldn't convince herself it had been a mistake. Eventually, the memory of just that blink of time when she had enjoyed something so special might be enough to persuade her that she was brave enough to try again. With someone who might want something more than a casual fling.

Maybe Pippa just needed to channel some of that masculine skill to separate sex and emotion.

Or she could follow the example of Sally, who'd gone through a string of brief relationships since she'd started working at Queen Mary's and they'd become good friends. Sally had even fallen head over heels in love a couple of times and had been devastated when the men had walked away, but she had the ability to bounce back. She wasn't even afraid of trying again.

Plenty more fish in the sea, she'd say. *One day I'll find a frog to kiss who actually does turn out to be a prince.*

She even had the ability to make a joke out of having a broken heart.

Time for another pity party with Pippa, she'd said last time. *And try saying that fast when you've had a wine or two.*

She might need a pity party herself, Pippa thought—complete with chocolate and wine and a weepy romantic movie—if she couldn't get how she was feeling about Lachlan under better control. She was dreading a case where she had to work closely with him again and her heart sank like a stone when Dawn Grimshaw arrived in the birthing suite. Pippa was the senior midwife on duty and Lachlan was the obstetrician on call and Dawn was going to need the most experienced staff members available. She was thirty-four weeks and three days pregnant—with triplets—and declared herself to be in established labour as she met Pippa by the reception desk.

Pippa was already very familiar with Dawn's history. She'd met this couple right at the start of the pregnancy, when Dawn had come in at eight weeks gestation, feeling ill, bleeding and convinced she was miscarrying her third child. She had been there when the stunned couple were given the news that three heartbeats had been found on the ultrasound examination.

Lachlan had already met Dawn as well. He'd

been on call when she had been admitted with a premature labour at almost thirty weeks. She had been given steroids to aid the babies' lung development but the other drugs administered had successfully stopped the labour so she'd been sent home again. It meant that Lachlan was familiar with Dawn's medical history and her determination to have a vaginal birth rather than a Caesarean and he would want to be involved with this delivery even if he wasn't on call.

'I'm sure it's the real thing this time,' Dawn said. 'The contractions are much stronger and longer and they're starting to hurt like hell.'

'The last ones have only been about three and a half minutes apart.' Dawn's husband, Graham, looked pale. 'I might have picked up a speeding ticket on the way here.'

'I kept my legs crossed,' Dawn said with a grimace. 'I also kept all my fingers crossed that Mr Smythe is in the building.'

'You're in luck,' Pippa said. 'He's not only in the building, he's on call. Rita? Could you bleep him, please? You'll find a plan in Dawn's notes for everyone else that needs to be called, too, like NICU and Paeds.'

Within a very short period of time, controlled chaos unfolded in the ward as a delivery suite was prepped, extra equipment was relocated, the neonatal intensive care unit was put on standby and additional paediatricians and midwives found to provide a team to care for each baby as it was born. Multiple births always created a buzz, especially when the mother wanted to avoid a surgical birth.

Lachlan appeared before anyone else, just as Pippa had got Dawn into the delivery suite and given her an initial assessment. It was Pippa's glance he caught first—just a graze of eye contact before greeting Dawn, but it was long enough for any misgivings she had about working with him to evaporate just as swiftly.

Personal feelings were totally irrelevant here. This was the man she wanted to work with. She might not trust him with her heart but she'd trust him with her life in an emergency and she had no qualms whatsoever trusting him to make sure these three identical boys arrived in the world safely.

'Dawn's five centimetres dilated,' she told Lachlan. 'Baby A cephalic. I'm about to set up the CTG and we've got a portable ultrasound on the way. Peter should be here any minute, and we've got Sally on standby for Baby B.'

Extra resuscitation units were being lined up to one side of the room to provide a space with oxygen, heating and light to assess a fragile newborn. They also had drawers full of the equipment, supplies and drugs that might be needed to fight for a tiny life.

'Who's Peter?' Dawn asked.

'He's one of our anaesthetists. I know how keen you are on having a completely natural birth, but remember how we talked about you having an epidural, just in case? It would be too late by the time you're fully dilated and there's a risk that, after the first baby is born, the others can turn into a more difficult presentation.'

Dawn's face was scrunching into lines of pain as another contraction began. 'I think I do want one. It's all very well when it's only one baby but this could go on for hours, couldn't it?' She groaned. 'Where's the consent form? I'll have to sign it, won't I?'

'Peter will have the forms with him,' Pippa said. 'But we've got the gas and air here if you want to use it now.' She turned on the Entonox cylinder valve, watched the needle of the pressure gauge rise to indicate that the tank was full and then got a clean mouthpiece from its packaging and clipped it onto the tubing before handing it to Dawn. The information she needed to pass on was automatic as she set the equipment up. 'This is for self-medication,' she said, 'so you need to hold the mouthpiece by yourself. Put it between your teeth and close your lips around it. When you feel the need for pain relief, breathe in deeply and only through your mouth. Pain relief should be rapid and any side-effects, like feeling dizzy or having tingling fingers, will wear off quickly as soon as you stop breathing it.'

Dawn sucked a deep breath in. And then another. She groaned again as she lay back on the pillows, this time in relief as the pain of the contraction faded. 'How long will an epidural take to start working?'

'It'll take about ten minutes to insert and another ten to fifteen minutes for the medication to take effect,' Lachlan responded. 'Peter will put a cannula in your hand as well and Pippa will put a bladder catheter in. We'll need to monitor the babies and your contractions, so we'll put two bands around your tummy for heartbeats and one for contractions and we'll use a scalp monitor for the baby that's arriving first. Are you okay with all this? I know you want things as natural as possible but it's my job to make sure it's as safe as possible.'

Dawn reached for her husband's hand and was holding it tightly as she nodded. 'We trust you,' she said.

Pippa looked up from where she was now unwinding the bands for the CTG monitor to see Peter coming into the room.

'Good timing,' she said. 'We were just talking about you.'

An hour later, the first triplet was delivered. A small but healthy baby boy who was pinking up and crying as his cord was clamped and cut. Dawn got to touch her baby for a moment before he was whisked into the care of the paediatric team and then taken to the neonatal intensive care unit.

'He weighs just under two kilograms,' Pippa relayed. 'That's four pounds two ounces in the old money. He's doing well.'

'Adam…' Graham's smile was proud but wobbly. 'That's what we're calling him.'

'Because he's Baby A,' Dawn added. 'It's Ben's turn next. Then Callum's.'

But Baby Ben wasn't in any hurry to appear. When Lachlan checked with both a physical examination and then the Doppler ultrasound, Pippa saw his expression change as he watched the images appear on screen.

'Ben seems to have taken advantage of the extra space Adam left in there.' His voice sounded as though this was no big deal but Pippa knew it could be. 'He's managed to turn into what's called a transverse position, which means he's lying sideways inside the uterus and, in his case, he's got his back to the door.'

'Oh, no… Does this mean I have to have a Caesarean now?' Dawn burst into tears.

'Not necessarily. I can try and turn him. If it

doesn't work from the outside, I can do an internal procedure. That means I put one hand inside the uterus and one hand on your tummy so I can shift baby enough to take hold of his legs and deliver him that way. If that's not successful, we have a theatre on standby and it will mean a Caesarean.'

'Please try,' Dawn sobbed. 'I don't want to go to Theatre.'

Pippa found she was holding her breath when the attempt to turn Baby B from the outside failed. An internal podalic version was a rare obstetric procedure and, while she knew what it entailed, she'd never seen one performed.

'You'll feel my hand inside,' Lachlan warned Dawn. 'But, with your epidural, it shouldn't be painful.'

His expression was one of intense concentration. He found the baby's head by palpating the outside of the belly and held it as he slipped his other hand into place to find the baby's feet and grasp them. Then both his hands were moving, gently but purposefully, shifting the baby so that he could be extracted. Pippa saw two tiny feet between Lachlan's fingers emerge and, only seconds later, baby Ben was taking his first breath. Again, his cord was clamped and cut, Dawn and Graham got a peek and the paediatric team took over.

He was bigger than Adam by a few ounces and, happily, his unusual entrance into the world didn't seem to have bothered him. They could all hear his loud protest as he was taken up to NICU to be with his brother.

Even more happily, the final triplet was in a perfect position and was delivered only fifteen minutes later. This time, with the neonatal consultant's approval, Pippa was able to hold the tiny baby for a little longer, letting his parents touch and kiss him before carrying him to the warmth of the resuscitation unit. And this time she wasn't focused on the babies still to be born and her role as Dawn's primary midwife. She could look down at this baby boy in her arms, wrapped in soft sterile towels.

She guessed he was pretty much the same weight as his brothers and he was breathing well but not crying. His eyes were open and it felt as if he was looking right back at Pippa. And he was so little…

And so perfect…

None of the babies that Pippa had miscarried had got anywhere near looking like this, but for some reason this felt exactly like how she'd imagined it would feel to finally hold a live baby of her own and her eyes suddenly filled with tears. Perhaps it was because there had been so many babies in her hands in such a short space of time. Or that things had been tense when Lachlan had dealt with what could have become a serious situation.

Or maybe it was because she'd been feeling oddly emotional ever since...

...ever since that night with Lachlan that was only a couple of weeks ago.

Since that dream when she'd realised how dangerously close she'd come to falling in love with him.

Oh, dear Lord...

Had he *felt* that thought?

Could he see tears that were on the point of escaping when he glanced in her direction at exactly the same moment she glanced in his?

Somehow, she found a smile. A kind of embarrassed one, as if she knew she was being less than professional by overreacting to the joy of a successful triplet delivery. It was good that she needed to turn away and hand the baby to the consultant. She stayed to watch as he assessed the third baby boy for his five-minute Apgar score because that gave her a moment or two to take a few deep breaths and centre herself.

By the time Dawn was through the last stage of her labour and could be taken to the NICU to finally meet her babies properly, Pippa found she was in a whole new headspace. She'd been through far worse things than a mild dose of heartbreak. Yes, there was a connection between herself and Lachlan but it probably wouldn't take any time at all for it to feel more like the bond of friendship she had with Sally.

As the days ticked past and it became apparent that Lachlan wasn't about to put any pressure on to make plans for another date, it felt as if the prospect had been put on a shelf—like a treat being kept for a special occasion?

If it was left there long enough to gather a bit of dust, Pippa thought, maybe it would be a mutual choice to simply forget about the still available third date and they could seamlessly pivot into being not only colleagues but real friends? That was, after all, the perfect ending when the mythical 'three date' rule was done and dusted, wasn't it? Lachlan would have no trouble at all finding someone who would be more than happy to have a friendship where those benefits weren't quite so limited.

Someone like Sally, perhaps, who came into the staffroom at the same time as Lachlan when Pippa was making herself a toastie for lunch.

'Have you heard?' she asked. 'That Lachlan's bought a house? In Richmond?'

'I had heard a rumour,' Pippa said cautiously. She kept her eye on the toasting machine to make sure Sally wouldn't see anything untoward in her face.

Pippa had been the first to know, hadn't she? Thank goodness nobody else knew that. Or that it was a house that had played its own part in what had happened between herself and Lachlan. She'd only bumped into him at the supermarket that day because he'd been to a viewing, and the day he'd put an offer in and it was accepted was the evening he'd come to that antenatal class she was running, with the tickets to the show that had been their second legitimate date. The one that couldn't be repeated because she'd discovered how close she'd come to falling in love with Lachlan.

She risked a quick glance at him. 'That's fantastic news. When do you move in?'

'It's a nice, quick settlement. I'll be in six weeks after the signing, so that's not far away now. Luckily, I've bought most of the furniture as well so I don't have to go on a mad shopping spree.'

'You are going to have a housewarming party, I hope.' Sally appeared from behind the fridge door, with her lunch container in her hands. 'And invite us all.' She grinned at Lachlan. 'Otherwise, our friendship might be over already.'

They all laughed, but Pippa still kept her gaze

on what she was doing as she extracted her sandwich from the machine.

A cheese sandwich.

Like the one she'd made for Lachlan on the night they'd first met.

The night when the air had been so full of those sparks of attraction. Pippa didn't feel very hungry any longer. Why hadn't she recognised the danger of those sparks? The fire they could ignite and how difficult it might be to hose down any hot spots?

'Oh…*wow*…' Sally's eyes widened dramatically. 'How lucky are you, Lachlan? To be waking up every morning to that *view*…'

Everybody was staring through the windows of the master bedroom, as Lachlan gave his guests a quick tour of his house.

Everybody except Pippa. From the corner of his eye, he'd caught the way she'd turned her head to flick a gaze in his direction—as if she couldn't help herself.

As if she was thinking the same thing he was. That they still had a date available and it could end up right here. In this room.

In this bed…

Lachlan broke the eye contact instantly. Before Pippa could see how much he wanted that date.

'That's exactly why I decided to buy this

place,' he told Sally. 'I've got a lot of happy childhood memories of Richmond Park.'

'It's a million-pound view, that's for sure.' But Peter was moving towards the walk-in wardrobe. 'No...you've got a dressing room *and* a full en-suite?'

'And four bedrooms?' Rita gave an audible sigh. 'I'm moving in, Lachlan.'

Pippa joined in the laughter, but she didn't catch his gaze again. Not that it stopped every cell in his body letting him know just how strong the longing was to make all these guests disappear and leave only himself and Pippa in this bedroom. Was it possible she might be the last to leave tonight?

'Come downstairs again,' he said. 'Let me get you all a drink and get this party really started.'

He led the way downstairs, hoping that getting well away from his bedroom would dampen the physical as well as the emotional reaction to seeing Pippa so close to his bed. Things had been going so well, too. Pippa hadn't put any pressure on to arrange that last permissible date in the game they'd been playing and she'd kept any hint of anticipation well-hidden at work, but surely she had to want it as much as he did? Who *wouldn't* want another night of the most sizzling but, at the same time, so exquisitely tender lovemaking that he was still feeling echoes from that night that were powerful enough to be disturbing, weeks after the experience.

Someone who was just as averse to hurting someone who might start wanting more than they were able to give?

It could also be someone who was afraid they might be hurt themselves because they were beginning to want more?

Either way, it seemed as if neither of them was willing to take the risk of cashing in that third date voucher. Lachlan would have to ignore the voice that had just begun whispering in the back of his head.

One more time couldn't hurt... The novelty might have worn off and it'll just be like sex with any other gorgeous woman...

Lachlan didn't think so.

'Help yourselves to anything you like.' He waved at the array of ice buckets and bottles on a sideboard in the drawing room. 'There's red and white wine and...prosecco of course. And champagne...' He was careful not to look in Pippa's direction as he popped the cork on a bottle. 'This is a celebration, after all. And it's my very first house-warming party.'

'Really?' Rita held a flute out to be filled. 'And you look like such a party animal, Mr Smythe.'

'It's the first house I've ever bought,' he told her.

'And you've chosen Richmond.' Sally also held out a glass. 'That's great. It must mean you're planning to stick around.'

'I guess so.' Lachlan raised an eyebrow in Pippa's direction, ready to fill a glass for her, but she gave her head a tiny shake and reached for a bottle of sparkling mineral water. Was this a signal that she didn't want to play? That she wouldn't still be here when all the other guests had departed later this evening?

Don't give up, that traitorous little voice suggested. *Try again later...with that special bottle of the vintage French champagne you've got in the fridge...*

Lachlan managed to find a smile for Sally. 'Maybe it was turning forty that made me decide it was time to settle down,' he said.

'Or it might be those childhood memories you can see out of your window,' Rita said. 'After all those years of globe-trotting, maybe you realised it was time to come home.' Her smile was warm as she raised her glass. 'Here's to coming home,' she toasted.

It seemed like everyone could think of something good to toast. Richmond. The park. The Queen Mary Hospital in general and the obstetric department in particular. Even wild swimming got thrown into the mix, along with laughter and a cheeky enquiry about whether bathing costumes were mandatory. Lachlan relaxed into being the host as it became clear that everyone was clearly enjoying the party.

He had plenty of snacks available but he'd arranged for hot pizzas to be delivered later in the evening that received an enthusiastic reception.

'This is perfect,' Peter said. 'I'm starving. Ooh…that one with anchovies has my name written all over it.' He picked up a large wedge with one hand and took a bite. He picked up the box with his other hand and held it out. 'Pippa?' His words were muffled by a full mouth. 'You've got to try this…'

Lachlan saw the moment that Pippa actually turned pale after she'd shaken her head and Peter had turned to offer the pizza to someone else. He watched her press her hand to her mouth seconds later, and then turn to run out of the room.

He felt his stomach dropping.

Something was wrong with Pippa.

The thought made him feel ill himself. He put down the piece of pizza he was holding and turned to follow Pippa out of the room, but Rita touched his arm.

'I'll go,' she said.

Lachlan had to nod. And smile. It was far more appropriate for motherly Rita to follow Pippa to the bathroom she had presumably headed for. The last thing Pippa would want would be for him to be showing a level of concern for her wellbeing that might be a giveaway for how well they knew each other.

It was several minutes before Rita came back.

'She's okay,' she told Lachlan. 'She just feels a bit off.'

'I hope it's not something she's eaten. Like those salmon canapés. What if I've given you all food poisoning?'

Rita patted his arm. 'Nobody else is feeling sick. Pippa said it was probably the smell of anchovies because she hates them with a passion, but I reckon she might have picked up that gastro bug that's going around. We had a toddler in Outpatients the other day who was throwing up all over the place.'

'Oh, no…'

'I'm going to take her home,' Rita told him. 'It's time I went and left you youngsters to enjoy yourselves anyway. Pippa said she doesn't want to make a fuss, so she asked me to pass on her thanks and that it's been a lovely party.'

The urge to stride out of the room and find Pippa so that he could see for himself that she really was okay was disturbingly powerful. Lachlan took a deep breath.

'Thanks for looking after her,' he said. 'Tell her I hope she feels better very soon.'

* * *

It had definitely been the anchovies.

Pippa felt quite well enough to go to work the day after Lachlan's housewarming party. She found some of her colleagues in the department's staffroom before handover was due to start. They were drinking what smelled like very strong coffee.

She grinned at Sally. 'So it was a good night, then?'

Sally nodded. 'You left early.'

'I wasn't feeling great. Me and anchovies don't get along.' She poured herself a mug of coffee and added milk.

'Ugh…' She glared at the mug after her first sip. 'Have we changed the brand of coffee or something? This tastes horrible.'

Sally laughed, reaching past her to rinse her mug and put it in the dishwasher. 'Tasted the same as always to me. Maybe you're pregnant.'

Pippa echoed her laughter. 'Yeah…right… Chance would be a fine thing.'

Sally's words came back to haunt her as she caught the first baby she delivered on that shift, however, lifting the baby girl to put her straight onto her mother's chest.

She'd never had any cravings in any of her pregnancies.

But she'd always gone off coffee. Big time.

It was impossible, of course. She was on the Pill and the chances of that form of contraception failing were only one percent.

Okay…the percentage went up if compliance wasn't perfect and Pippa did miss the occasional dose.

There'd been the issue of the broken condom too, but that was how many weeks ago? Seven? Eight? She would have had signs by now, even if the Pill had made her periods light enough to be barely noticeable sometimes.

Signs like going off coffee?

Throwing up at the smell of anchovies?

There were pregnancy tests freely available in the ward and, just to reassure herself, Pippa took one with her when she went for a bathroom break late that afternoon when her shift was over. She stayed in the cubicle, sitting on the toilet and staring at the little window on the stick for the three minutes it took to develop.

It didn't take three minutes, though. Clearly, she was excreting enough HCG hormone for the test line to develop almost as quickly and strongly as the control line. There was no doubt about it.

Pippa was pregnant.

CHAPTER NINE

'ARE YOU OKAY, Pippa? You look a bit pale.'

'Yeah…all good, thanks, Rita. Just a bit tired.' Pippa kept walking. Out of the ward and out of Queen Mary's.

She'd been lying, of course. She wasn't okay. The last thing she'd expected—or wanted—was to find herself pregnant.

Again.

To be facing the pain, both physical and emotional, of losing yet another baby. Which would happen within the next few weeks, given how far along she was already. She'd never got past the first trimester. Sometimes it had been only days after a positive test that the bottom fell out of her world yet again.

Thanks to assuming her ultra-light periods were due to the contraceptive pill, she had to be only a couple of weeks away from the end point of her first trimester so she had every reason to suspect that the cramps and bleeding would start any day now.

Which meant that there was really no point in telling Lachlan that she was pregnant, was there?

Especially when it would ruin the friendship that seemed to be growing between them—the perfect common ground that would never derail her life in the way that falling in love with someone who was unavailable could have done.

She could hear his voice so clearly as she walked home that evening, telling her that he liked rules about dating. That he had a few of his own.

Like keeping things strictly casual. That's non-negotiable...

Casual. It would be unacceptable for someone to fall in love with him. Or to dream of a committed relationship or, heaven forbid, marriage or children.

Non-negotiable.

Nobody was ever going to persuade him to change his mind.

She'd been lucky to get as close to Lachlan as she had. Pippa had the feeling that it would be a rare privilege to be considered a good friend.

Falling pregnant had broken every rule Lachlan Smythe had about dating.

If she told him, he would never trust her again and they could never be friends.

She'd been through this herself often enough to know that she would survive. Doing it alone, in fact, would be preferable to the support of her ex-husband and the obstetrician who'd actually been sleeping with him at the time of her last miscarriage.

Pippa couldn't even tell Sally because if any hint got out, it could get back to Lachlan and he knew she hadn't been seeing anyone else. He would be able to add lying by omission to any other aspects of what would seem like a betrayal. He might even think that she'd been lying about being on the Pill.

By the time Pippa had arrived home at her little cottage, she was exhausted by overthinking everything. It was really quite simple. All she needed to do was to stay calm and carry on. This problem would be history within a matter of only a few days. Weeks, at the very most.

Whatever bug had targeted Pippa on the night of his housewarming party seemed to be having long-lasting effects. She certainly wasn't looking a hundred percent. She was still a little pale a week later and she seemed…subdued?

Not her usual self, that was for sure.

She was, however, still smiling and still caring for her mothers with the same focus and skill Lachlan had come to expect from her.

She'd called for obstetric assistance this morning and her summary was succinct.

'I have a thirty-six-year-old primigravida who's been in second stage labour for nearly three hours and getting very tired. We now have a non-reassuring CTG with a baseline heart rate between one hundred and one-oh-five and variable decelerations over the last twenty minutes or so that are lasting more than sixty seconds and are biphasic.'

'I'm on my way,' Lachlan said.

The CTG recordings were even more concerning by the time Lachlan arrived in the birthing suite and suggested that the level of oxygen the baby was receiving was not ideal.

'On the plus side,' Lachlan said, after explaining why Pippa had called for assistance, 'I know you feel too tired to carry on pushing but your contractions still have a good duration and intensity, which means you'll be able to help us if we try some assistance with either a vacuum cup or forceps.'

After a physical examination he told her that it might be as simple as correcting the position of the baby's head. 'Your baby could be born within a few minutes,' he said. 'If we go for a Caesarean, even though you've got an epidural in place, it'll take quite a lot more time to get you up to Theatre and prepped for surgery. And the less time it takes, the better that is for baby, when oxygen levels might be dropping.'

The frightened first-time parents listened to the risk factors for both the procedure and the back-up plan for a C-section if it failed. He saw them both look to Pippa for reassurance.

'Mr Smythe is the best possible obstetrician you could have,' she told them, the sincerity in her tone completely genuine. 'If this was my baby, I'd absolutely trust him to choose the safest option for his birth.'

Within minutes, the consent form was signed. Peter arrived to top up the epidural anaesthetic and Sally arrived to assist Pippa.

'Paediatrics are caught up in Theatre and ED,' Peter reported. 'Someone will be here asap.'

Lachlan scrubbed in and got gowned and gloved. He could see that Pippa and Sally were both busy, getting the mother into position with her legs in stirrups, draping her legs and belly and inserting a catheter to make sure her bladder was empty. A trolley appeared beside him with all the equipment he needed.

He checked the gear, putting the cup of the vacuum device against his palm and pumping it to make sure it was functioning correctly and the vacuum pressure would hold. He carefully palpated the baby's skull, finding the triangular shape of the posterior fontanelle and the diamond shape of the anterior fontanelle near the forehead. He positioned the cup over the midline between the fontanelles. Looking up, he found Pippa's steady gaze on his and he gave her a single nod.

She was keeping a close eye on the CTG screen.

'Here it comes, Anika… Are you ready? Deep breath in and push. Push…push…push— You're doing *great*.'

Lachlan was applying gentle traction on the baby's head.

'Take another deep breath.' Pippa was taking one herself as if she was sharing this part of the labour with the mother. 'And…push…push… *push…*'

The top of the baby's head was visible as the contraction faded. They waited for the next one to start and Pippa was even more encouraging.

'Push as hard as you can. This one will do it. Push hard. *Harder…* You're almost there…'

Lachlan changed the direction of his traction to pull the head up. With his other hand he felt under the baby's face and as soon as he could feel the jaw he released the suction cap.

'Your baby's head is born, Anika,' he said. 'You can push his body out now.'

'One more,' Pippa said. 'Just one more push…'

And there he was. He heard Pippa's intake of breath as she noticed how limp and blue the baby was. Lachlan immediately clamped and cut the cord and Pippa scooped the infant into a sterile towel and took him straight to the resuscitation unit. The paediatric team still hadn't arrived. Sally took over monitoring Anika for the third stage of her labour.

'What's happening?' Anika cried. 'What's wrong?'

'Baby just needs a little bit of help,' Lachlan told her. He stripped off his gloves and was pulling on a fresh pair as he joined Pippa. The baby boy was dry and in the warmth of the unit. Oxygen was flowing and Pippa had a tiny mask over his face and was helping him with his first breaths. Lachlan could already see that the blue tinge to his skin was fading and he was moving—tiny arms and legs beginning to wake up. The disc of Lachlan's stethoscope covered half the little chest but what he could hear made him smile.

'Heart rate's over a hundred,' he told Pippa.

She lifted the mask and the baby took his first breath on his own. And then another that came with a warbling cry as it was released.

'Apgar of two at one minute,' Pippa said quietly. 'Up to seven at five minutes.'

'Can we see him?' Anika called. *'Please…?'*

Lachlan caught Pippa's gaze and gave her another single nod. She wrapped the baby in a fresh warm towel and gathered him into her arms to take to his parents. Lachlan found he was watching her rather than the baby so he saw the moment she had to blink back tears as she picked up the baby. It was then he remembered her reaction at the birth of the triplets last week, but this time he could sense an intensity that was…

…different, that was what it was.

But both those births had come with the kind of tension where a tiny life was potentially hanging in the balance. It was normal to feel the kind of relief that could bring a lump to your throat or a tear to your eye.

What was making him think that there was something more going on with Pippa? Making him feel as if he wanted to find out what it was. To ask for that third date so they could have a really private conversation? Pillow talk, even, where secrets could be shared?

No. That would be a bad idea. A really, really bad idea.

What he could do, though, was keep a careful eye on her and make sure she was okay. Because what if it had been something he'd done, or hadn't done, that had changed things? That it was his fault she was more emotional about her job and that she looked…almost haunted?

* * *

The twelve-week mark for the pregnancy finally arrived.

Then a few more days went past—so slowly that Pippa felt as if she was counting every single minute.

She'd never got this far in a pregnancy.

She'd never felt this…*good*…

That nausea was gone. She had more energy. And, from somewhere she couldn't control, Pippa began to feel flickers of…not hope exactly, but the first acknowledgement that maybe this time might be different.

That this, in fact, could turn out to be what she'd always dreamed of—the journey to becoming a mother. It kind of made sense. The father was different this time. Perhaps there had been some kind of chemical incompatibility in every one of those earlier pregnancies that wasn't there this time.

It was still far too early to be confident, of course. It was hard enough to believe she'd got this far. Maybe that was why, when the department was so quiet, late in her shift that day, Pippa decided to drink a large glass of water to fill her bladder, wait half an hour and then sneak into an unoccupied room and use the ultrasound machine—just to prove to herself that she really was still pregnant.

She angled the screen of the machine so that she could see it from the bed, propped herself up on pillows, pulled the elastic waistband of her scrub pants down and squirted gel onto her belly. Then she slid the transducer as low as she could and pressed it into the midline, angling it down to locate her bladder right behind her pubic bone. She held her breath as she changed the angle to find the uterus that was right beside the bladder and...

...and there it was. The dark fluid in her uterus and the unmistakable shape of a baby. She could see the head that looked too big and even identify tiny limbs. Legs that were actually *kicking*...

And the soft swish of a foetal heartbeat was filling the air.

'Oh, my God...' she whispered.

Pippa was overwhelmed. So focused on the screen and the rhythmic swishing she was oblivious to anything else, including the sound of the door being quietly opened and then clicked shut again.

She jumped, gripping the transducer more tightly at the sound of a voice in the darkened room.

'What the hell is going on in here?'

Pippa gasped. Of all the people who could

have discovered what she was doing, this was the worst possible contender.

'*Lachlan…?*'

She couldn't move. The transducer was still on her belly. The image was still filling the screen. Lachlan walked towards the machine, sat down in front of it and reached for the transducer. Pippa's fingers went limp enough to let him take hold of the handle.

'I saw you coming in here,' he said, his tone expressionless. 'When you didn't come out, I started to wonder whether you were okay.'

Pippa could feel the pressure of the transducer on her belly deepen. She could see that Lachlan knew exactly what he was doing. He used the callipers to click on the frozen image of the baby, putting a marker on the tip of the head and another one on the rump. With the second click, a dotted line appeared and she knew that the machine was calculating the crown to rump length to provide a gestational age.

Lachlan was completely silent as he looked at the information. He changed the angle of the transducer and did a sideways sweep.

'Singleton pregnancy,' he said finally. 'Gestational age of twelve weeks, five days—give or take four days for accuracy.' His voice was just a monotone. It was icy. 'Is it mine?'

'Yes…' The word was a whisper. 'I'm sorry.'

Except she wasn't. Not now. Not when she could see this new life that had been created. When she could still hear that heartbeat.

But Lachlan lifted the transducer and the sound stopped. He sat there, the light of the screen making his face look ghostly. Frozen. He was sitting very still and the silence was deadly. Unbearable.

Pippa picked up a paper towel to scrub the gel off her belly. She needed to get out of here.

Lachlan turned the machine off and the screen went dark. He said only five words.

'You can't have this baby.'

The shock was electric. Pippa could feel it all over her skin—a horrible, prickling sensation. Sinking in to make her feel sick and create a weird buzzing in her head.

She was moving without giving her body any conscious instructions. Screwing up the paper towel. Pulling her scrub pants back up and swinging her legs off the bed.

She threw six words over her shoulder as her feet touched the floor.

'That's not your choice to make.'

And then she walked out of the room.

CHAPTER TEN

IT WASN'T A conscious choice to stay there staring at that black screen after Pippa had stormed out of the room.

It was simply that Lachlan couldn't move.

This was a body blow he hadn't seen coming. Even when he was going through the motions of clicking the cursor and taking the measurements that would reveal the gestational age of this unborn baby and it was sinking in that it could be *his* baby, he still hadn't seen this coming.

Something that was so huge, his world could never be the same.

It only lasted a heartbeat, but that was enough.

Enough for Lachlan to come face to face with something he'd managed to bury so deeply he hadn't even known it existed.

The strength of that longing to have a family of his own.

To be a husband. To be a father. To live, like most people could, without the fear of an unimaginably horrible disease becoming a reality—for a parent, for yourself or, even worse, for your child.

The fear was always going to win over any longing, of course, but that glimpse of what it could have been like had been the most painful blow Lachlan had experienced in too many years to count.

He'd seen the baby. Not just a shapeless blob with only the astonishing evidence of life that a tiny beating heart represented. Pippa's pregnancy was so far along that the outline of limbs was now clear, right down to minuscule fingers and toes. The button of a nose, the curl of developing ears. That was what had made the longing so fierce. And the fear so very real.

He'd had to hit back. It was self-defence. A shield that he pulled in front of himself. He hadn't intended that his words would come out as starkly as they had. Or as such a blunt commandment.

You can't have this baby...

Pippa had been perfectly correct in stating that it wasn't his choice to make. What she didn't know was that she wasn't making an informed choice herself. She had no idea of how much pain and suffering could be in her future. Or the child's. Or *his*, for that matter, which felt unfair when he'd been so determined—and careful— to make sure that this would never happen. That he would never have to go back into the space where he knew exactly what it would be like to live with the threat of Huntington's in the background of every minute of every day. A space he'd managed to lock the door on years ago. A space that he'd never the slightest inclination to re-enter.

Pippa had unlocked that door.

She hadn't given him any choice about going back in there either, because she'd *pushed* him in.

The longing was forgotten. Even the fear was fading. It was kind of like a game of emotional rock-paper-scissors.

Fear squashed hope. But anger could beat fear.

Lachlan could finally move again.

Okay, his words had been too harsh, given that Pippa did not know what had prompted them.

He owed her an explanation.

But he couldn't do that while he was feeling like this. The anger was another type of shield, and somehow he needed to find the courage to put it down before he would be able to speak to her.

It was the fastest U-turn Pippa Gordon had ever made.

Hopefully fast enough that the man at the other end of the corridor—Lachlan Smythe—

hadn't seen her change direction in a very blatant attempt to avoid crossing his path.

She turned the corner at the end of the corridor and went into the first room she had access to, which was an unoccupied delivery suite. This was supposed to be her lunch break but Pippa had just completely lost her appetite. She needed to find a distraction and she could see one right in front of her. A neonatal resuscitation unit. It wouldn't hurt to double-check this vital piece of equipment and make sure nothing was missing from any of the external or internal components.

She flicked the switch to turn it on and check that the heater and lights were functioning. Then she checked that the oxygen and air cylinders were full and there were no signs of wear and tear on the hoses.

Her concentration slipped as she counted the towels and linen, however.

If she had to work with Lachlan, fine. She could deal with that, but Pippa had no intention of talking to him if she could avoid it and it wasn't anything other than a strictly professional conversation. She didn't even want to say hello to him.

She opened the first drawer under the bassinet mattress within its clear plastic walls. This was where the infant laryngoscopes were slotted, along with blades and introducers. There were the smallest sized plastic airways, too. And nasogastric tubes. They were all so miniature. The fight for newborn babies' lives was not just incredibly tense, it was so much more delicate because their airways and veins and arteries were so tiny and fragile.

How *dared* Lachlan tell her she couldn't have this baby?

Nobody was going to tell her what she could or couldn't do when it came to her body.

She was still furious, three days after he'd busted her giving herself an ultrasound examination.

Pippa took a deep breath as she opened another drawer and used her expert gaze to scan for any gaps in a wide range of supplies. Cannulas and bandages and splints. Syringes and needles and clamps and dressings. Every compartment of the drawer seemed to be well stocked and she finally let her breath out in a sigh.

Oh, she'd known Lachlan wouldn't react well to the news. He'd told her straight up that he was 'on board' with her assumed aversion to any long-term relationship that even resembled a marriage, and being linked to someone through parenthood was about as long-term as it got.

He had been amused enough to suggest that he was totally on board with her opinion that the old woman who lived in a shoe was 'stupid' because she had so many children. He'd laughed aloud. And making him laugh had added fuel to the fire of that instant attraction, hadn't it?

It didn't seem very funny now, though.

Okay…so he was the father of this baby. That gave him the right to know of its existence. To be part of its life if he chose to be, but it didn't give him the right to choose whether this baby was born or not. If he didn't want any part of being a father, well, that was fine, too. Pippa could cope perfectly well as a single mother, just like millions of other women managed to do.

Had she really thought he wouldn't have noticed her?

Lachlan had been aware that Pippa was doing her best to avoid him. He'd been doing the same thing himself in order to try and clear his own head, but seeing her practically running away so that she didn't have to walk past him was unacceptable. It was so blatant, people were going to notice. And start asking questions.

They hadn't had to work together closely in the last three days, largely thanks to him having a day off and some back-to-back meetings, but what was going to happen when they did? Was she going to turn around and walk away from a mother who needed assistance with a forceps delivery? Or stand at one side of the theatre, her body posture radiating hostility, while he performed an emergency Caesarean?

Lachlan had lengthened his stride, but by the time he reached the end of the corridor Pippa was nowhere to be seen in either direction and he didn't have time to stand there wondering how he was going to deal with this situation. He was due to start an outpatient clinic for high-risk pregnancies due to medical conditions.

There were women waiting for him who were desperate to have a child, despite the extra risk of congenital heart malformations, high blood pressure, renal failure or brittle diabetes. Brave women who deserved his complete concentration and best efforts to keep the pregnancy safe for as long as possible and ensure that both mother and baby stayed healthy.

His first patient was already waiting in the consulting room and Lachlan picked up her notes as he went past the reception desk, pushing Pippa Gordon and *her* pregnancy completely out of his mind until the rest of his working day was finished.

Anna was a Type One diabetic and while she'd been managing her blood sugar levels well during her pregnancy, the complication of excess amniotic fluid had been noted at her last visit so she was being monitored more closely now.

'How are you feeling, Anna?'

'Not too bad. I'm getting a bit short of breath if I walk too far. Or do the vacuuming or something.'

Anna's husband, Clint, was smiling as they exchanged a fond glance. 'That's her excuse, anyway. I'm getting very good at vacuuming.'

'Have you noticed any swelling in your legs or feet?'

'No.'

'Indigestion? Heartburn?'

'Yes—but that's par for the course at this stage of pregnancy now, isn't it? I'm thirty-six weeks.'

Lachlan was scanning the report from the ultrasound examination Anna had just had. 'There's quite an increase in the amount of fluid from your last visit. Come and get up on the couch so I can have a feel of your tummy.'

Anna used the step to get onto the examination couch. Clint helped her get comfortable by rearranging the pillows and she glanced over to where Lachlan was washing his hands as she settled back.

'Is it dangerous?' she asked. 'It feels like we should be really worried with all these extra appointments.'

'We just want to keep a close eye on you, which is why we're getting you to come in so often. There is an increased risk of a premature birth or the baby being able to turn and become a breech presentation and we have to be aware of other potential complications like a cord prolapse or part of the placenta becoming detached.'

Clint nodded. 'Our midwife gave us a list of everything to watch out for and she told us not to hesitate to come in and get checked if we're worried about anything. She's really lovely. Pippa Gordon, her name is. Do you know her?'

'I do indeed.' Lachlan nodded as he reached for some paper towels. 'She's a wonderful midwife.'

For a split second, as Lachlan dried his hands thoroughly, his focus slipped. He could so easily imagine Pippa making sure someone like Anna was fully informed and she would know what she was talking about as far as risk factors to either baby or mother. If she didn't know enough about something like polyhydramnios, she would do whatever research was needed to get up to speed.

Was that the problem with this stand-off they were in?

Just giving her the bare facts, as he'd intended to do, and explaining that going ahead with a pregnancy was unacceptable if a test confirmed the risk of Huntington's Disease might well not be enough for Pippa.

She deserved to hear the whole story.

Even if that didn't change how she felt about

the situation she had the right to know the risks she would be facing in the future. It was a moral duty on his part to make sure that she *was* fully informed, however hard that was going to be.

He'd finally reached a stage in his life where he'd found a very welcome peace. Where he could experience a memory, like bike riding with Liam, that could bring joy rather than push him back into the space where the worst of the other memories had been filed and locked away.

Telling Pippa everything could risk undermining this new peace so much that he might never find it again. But he had no choice, did he?

Pippa deserved an explanation.

She also deserved an apology for what he'd said to her.

Not that she was going to let him get close enough to have any kind of conversation at work, and that would be entirely inappropriate for the extremely personal discussion he intended having with her. She was just as unlikely to accept an invitation from him to meet somewhere else, so there was really only one solution. He would simply have to turn up on her doorstep and force her to listen to him.

And there was something else he would have to do first.

Something that would have to wait until this clinic was completed and he was satisfied that there was nothing he needed to do urgently to keep all these high-risk mothers and babies safe.

'Let's get started,' he said aloud, screwing up the paper towels and dropping them into the wastepaper basket. 'Did you have a BGL finger prick when you went for your blood tests earlier?'

'No. They mentioned things like renal and liver function. I do have an appointment at the diabetes clinic in a couple of days. I am noticing that my insulin levels need adjusting more often at the moment, which is a bit of a pain.'

'I'll test it now, if you're okay with that. I'd just like to double-check it against your continuous monitor for accuracy.'

'No problem.'

Anna held her finger out to get a drop of blood collected. Then Lachlan wrapped a blood pressure cuff around her upper arm. He was going to do a thorough obstetric check-up and had set aside plenty of time to explain the possibility of inducing labour earlier—possibly as early as next week if the baby kept growing this fast. The need for a C-section was another possibility that they needed to be aware of.

His patient after Anna was Caitlin, who'd had a congenital heart defect corrected as a child and was now also well into her third trimester. The final couple he saw needed extra time simply to reassure them, not only because they were expecting twins, and multiple pregnancies were automatically higher risk and therefore received more frequent monitoring. This couple had been trying to get pregnant for more than ten years and had finally achieved success thanks to IVF treatment in another city. They were understandably highly anxious so it was much later than normal business hours by the time they left, but Lachlan had a phone number that he knew he could use to make this particular call.

The person he spoke to was a very senior doctor at London's Regional Genetics Centre—one of the specialist services for the diagnosis and management of genetic conditions.

'Of course I remember you, Lachlan. And your family.' His tone was gentle. 'What can I do for you today?'

'I'm ready,' was all Lachlan had to say. 'Could I possibly make an appointment to come and see you tomorrow?'

CHAPTER ELEVEN

IT HAD BEEN a long day.

Eighteen-year-old Kayley, who'd become pregnant accidentally and had no intention of keeping her baby and no desire to go through the process of giving birth, had come in with regular contractions that had continued for several hours with little progress. The atmosphere in the room was tense and miserable, which wasn't helping anyone.

'The gas isn't working. I want an epidural.'

'You're not quite dilated enough to have an epidural yet.' Pippa had estimated it to be barely two centimetres on last examination. 'We need to be sure you're in established labour. If things don't get going again, we might need to send you home for a while and we can't do that if you've had an epidural.'

'I don't want to go home. I want a Caesarean.'

'You really don't, Kayley. Not unless it's really necessary. It's major surgery that can be very painful afterwards and it takes a long time to recover. Let's get you up and walking around. That might help.'

'You'll be lucky.' Kayley's mother was flicking through a magazine as she sat beside the bed. 'It's hard enough getting this one out of bed on a good day.'

'Would you like me to get one of the doctors to come and see you, Kayley?' Pippa sent a silent wish into the ether that it wasn't Lachlan on call today. His days off had overlapped hers and she wasn't sure if he was even back in the hospital yet. She wasn't feeling nearly as angry as she had been, but she was still hoping to avoid working with him for as long as possible.

'What for?' Kayley muttered.

'To talk about options for pain relief. Or helping to get your labour established.' Beneath the surliness and lack of cooperation, Pippa could see the teenager's fear. 'I know this isn't easy for you, sweetheart,' she said gently. 'We all want to help.'

'Do what the nurse says, Kay.' Her mother dropped the magazine. 'I'm going home for a bit to see what chaos your brothers are creating but I'll be back later, okay?'

'Whatever...' Kayley picked up the Entonox mouthpiece and dragged in a deep breath. Then she dropped it over the side of the bed. 'It's *still* not working. It's useless...'

It turned out to be Sandy on call and she was brilliant with Kayley. She made the teenager feel as if she was taking some control of the situation as they made a plan to break her waters, start an oxytocin drip and get an epidural in place sooner rather than later.

Six long, hard hours later, an exhausted Kayley was holding her baby in her arms, and Pippa's heart was squeezed hard at the pride in this young mother's face.

'Look at him, Mum...'

'Yeah...he's pretty cute. You don't want to keep him now, do you?'

'I dunno... This doesn't feel like I thought it was going to.'

'You don't have to make any big decisions yet,' Pippa said. 'The whole team will be in tomorrow with all the people you need to talk to, like your counsellors and psychologist and social worker. It's time to rest now. You've done a brilliant job, Kayley. You should be very proud of yourself.'

Kayley smiled at her for the first time since she'd arrived this morning. 'I guess I am. Well tired, though.'

Pippa was well tired herself. She got home, kicked her shoes off, opened the door of the fridge to see what she had available to cook for dinner and then pushed it shut again. Cooking was a step too far. Her phone was in the pocket of her coat hanging by the front door. After a day like today, she deserved to order something hot that would be delivered, hopefully before she fell asleep on the couch.

The knock on her door as she reached into the coat pocket made her jump. Opening the door to find someone standing there with paper bags that were clearly full of takeout food was nothing short of a miracle.

The only problem was that the person holding the bags was Lachlan.

'We need to talk,' he said quietly. 'Can I come in, please?' He lifted the bags. 'I come with food. Did you know *Chez Anton* caters for takeout? I thought you might let me in if I brought posh steak and chips.'

Oh-h...

He was smiling at her and for a moment Pippa was pulled back to that dream she'd had. The one when she'd been so devastated when he walked away from her and it felt as if her world had shattered.

She'd had her suspicions then that she might have already fallen in love with him and, while she'd dismissed it, it was more than a suspicion at the moment. But she was overtired. Pregnant and hormonal. He had arrived with hot, deli-cious-smelling food and he was smiling at her.

Caring for her…

What woman wouldn't fall in love with a man like this?

She was too tired to even try and summon the shock and anger she'd had at his reaction to finding out that she was pregnant with his baby.

She tried. She tried to remind herself that she preferred the idea of being a single mother to having anything to do with Lachlan Smythe ever again. She opened her mouth to tell him to go away and leave her alone. But she found herself saying something rather different.

'You'd better come in then,' she said.

He'd even brought sparkling mineral water for her to replace the champagne they'd had to ac-company exactly this meal they'd had on their first date. Oddly, it felt even more delicious to be curled up on the couch, still in her scrubs, with bare feet, eating the crispy twice-cooked fries and slivers of steak with her fingers. She knew Lachlan wanted to talk but they ate in a com-panionable silence with nothing more important being said than how perfectly cooked the food was and how good was tarragon and chervil to-gether in a sauce?

But then the meal was over, the containers piled back into the paper bags and their fingers wiped on the serviettes that had come with the meals. Pippa found herself curling further back into the corner of her sofa. Lachlan leaned forward, his hands on his knees and his head bent. He let his breath out slowly.

'I need to tell you a story,' he said.

'Okay…' There was something in Lachlan's tone that tugged at her heartstrings enough to make her want to reach out and touch him. To reassure him?

To let him know that she could care for him the way he'd just shown he could care for her?

Whatever it was, Pippa resisted it. She hugged her arms around herself instead. Around her belly and the baby she needed to protect.

'I had a younger brother,' Lachlan said quietly. 'His name was Liam and he was three years younger than me. By the time I was five, he was old enough to be fun to play with and I was his favourite person in the world. He'd be waiting for me at the gate when I got home from school with some awful present like a soggy, half-eaten biscuit he'd saved for me and…' he cleared his throat '…and I loved him so much that I'd eat it and pretend it was the best present ever.'

Lachlan didn't lift his head so he didn't see that Pippa was smiling. She knew that kind of love that could exist between siblings.

'He was so excited when he started school,

but that was when people noticed that something wasn't right. He was a bit clumsier than the other kids and sometimes he walked oddly. One of his teachers said he looked like a little old man. She thought it was cute, but what did worry her was his learning problems. They did all sorts of educational tests and thought he might have ADHD. He got sessions with a psychologist and a speech therapist.'

Pippa was listening quietly. Watching Lachlan. She could feel his pain even though his voice sounded perfectly normal. Calm. In control. The way he was with patients when he was taking charge of a potential emergency. Exactly the skilled professional you wanted to be in charge, and that meant keeping an emotional distance so that his focus couldn't be derailed.

'He had a seizure one day at school and that took things to another level. He was given an MRI and they suspected Huntington's Disease.'

Pippa's inward breath was a gasp. 'In a *child*?'

Lachlan turned his head just enough to give her a graze of eye contact. 'It's rare but it happens. They call it "The Devil's Disease"—the cruellest disease known to man.'

Pippa swallowed the huge lump in her throat. She didn't want to hear any more of this story.

But she couldn't *not* hear the rest of it.

'My parents got tested and my father had a

positive result for the disease. He was already well into his forties so he knew he was likely to start getting symptoms by the time he was fifty, but he refused to talk about it. It was Liam that mattered. His son. The child he was supposed to protect, and it was his fault that he now had this terrible disease. I remember seeing him cry for the first time. And seeing him look at me as if he was wondering whether he was going to lose both his sons before he died himself.'

Pippa could actually feel the blood draining from her face. Had Lachlan been tested? Was he working up to tell her that he also had Huntington's and therefore the baby she was carrying had a fifty percent chance of having inherited the genetic disorder? It had to be. She could still hear the hollow tone of his voice, as if she was doing something completely unthinkable.

You can't have this baby...

Lachlan threw another glance at Pippa, as if he'd guessed what she might be thinking but he wasn't ready to answer that unspoken question yet.

'Liam's seizures became more and more frequent,' he continued quietly. 'In general, the younger the child is when the symptoms appear, the shorter time they survive, and the progression was rapid for Liam—only ten years from diagnosis. I was eighteen. Liam was fifteen.'

Pippa closed her eyes. 'I'm so sorry, Lachlan,' she whispered.

'It was my mother I was most sorry for in the end,' he said. 'She had devoted her life to caring for Liam. Both she and Dad were devastated when he died and…and we thought that Dad's depression was part of his grief. Until the other symptoms began to appear. I was lucky. They wouldn't hear of me not going away to university and then medical school. The progression of the disease could take decades. It didn't, but it still took too long before my mother finally admitted she couldn't cope with caring for him at home. He spent his last year in a home, unable to talk or move or even swallow. He was still the centre of Mum's life. She visited him every single day and…when he died, she just seemed to fade away. Her official cause of death was a heart attack. It's not very scientific, but I believe it was more like a broken heart.'

Pippa had tears rolling down her cheeks.

She had to touch Lachlan, and when she reached towards him he took hold of her hand, gave it a squeeze, but then let it go. He wasn't finished. Pippa took a deep breath. He was going to tell her what she desperately needed to know. She couldn't let the breath out until he did.

'They didn't test me as a child,' Lachlan said. 'Unless you're symptomatic they won't do it until you're eighteen and can choose for yourself. I'd seen what Liam went through and I didn't want to know if it was going to happen to me, so I chose not to get tested. I watched what happened to my father and my mother, who didn't even have the disease, and that only confirmed that I'd made the right decision for myself.'

Pippa had to let her breath out, but it wasn't a sigh of relief. She still didn't know. Fear was digging its claws in.

'It's the toss of a coin.' Lachlan shrugged. 'Heads, you're fine. You can live a normal life. Tails, you're facing a degenerative, life-threatening brain disease and life will never be normal again. I preferred to live with the hope I might be free of it.' He let his breath out in a sigh. 'I knew if I got symptomatic I'd have no choice but to face it and I was okay with that. Because I would be doing it by myself. I wouldn't have a partner that would have to live through it and have their own life ruined like my mother's was. Above all, I was going to make damned sure I never risked passing it on to a child because I felt that was a social responsibility as well as a personal one. The only way, so far, to eradicate the disease is to stop passing it on. And yes, I could have found a partner and tested embryos and terminated pregnancies that were affected, but how could I willingly give my partner and healthy kids the prospect of having to live with me when it was my turn and I knew how horrendous it would be?'

Lachlan got to his feet. He turned and, for the first time, he made direct eye contact with Pippa. And held it.

'I've had the test now. It could take weeks to get the results, but if I'm negative there won't be any repercussions for the baby.'

Pippa was holding her breath as well as Lachlan's gaze.

If he was negative, wouldn't that mean that there was no longer a reason for Lachlan to fear letting anyone close enough to him to be swept up into the horror of watching him slowly die? No reason for him not to have his own family and be a father?

But the grim tone of Lachlan's voice was more than enough to warn her that it was far too soon to go anywhere near that kind of hope.

'If I'm not negative,' he continued, 'prenatal testing is available through amniocentesis from fourteen to eighteen weeks, but that's an ethical minefield we can discuss if it turns out to be necessary.'

Oh… *God*…

Pippa had done this.

She'd pushed Lachlan into a space where he had to face his worst nightmare. When any hope of living a normal life without the fear of this dreadful disease could be taken away from him. They might both have to live with the fear that their child could be affected. She cared deeply about this man and *she* had done this to him.

Pippa's overwhelming emotions must have been written all over her tear-streaked face because she saw the tight lines of Lachlan's face soften a little.

'I'm sorry I told you that you couldn't have this baby,' he said. 'I had no right to say that. But now you know why I said it.'

She could see the muscles of his throat moving as he swallowed. Hard. Was *he* trying not to cry? Did he need to escape? Was that why he was already heading towards the door?

The urge to follow and put her arms around him was so strong, Pippa could feel herself starting to move and it was in that moment that she realised how much she loved Lachlan.

How much she wanted to be with him—for better *or* worse.

But she also understood how impossible that was.

Lachlan was never going to let anyone that close.

Ironically, the more he cared about someone the less likely he would be to want to spend time with them, let alone make a lifetime commitment. The more he cared, the more effort he would put in to sparing them having to potentially watch someone *they* loved suffer so much.

She'd gone an even bigger step further into the forbidden territory of relationships. She was the person who'd forced him to break a vow and risk the worst thing he could imagine doing in his life—passing on an unthinkable future to an innocent child.

Even if going through this testing ended up releasing him from the fear of letting someone get close enough to create a family with, maybe it wouldn't be with *her*, because she'd done something so cruel to him.

'I'm sorry, too,' she whispered.

But Lachlan didn't hear her. The door was already closing behind him.

CHAPTER TWELVE

'HOW ARE YOU FEELING, Anna?'

'I'm okay... I think...'

Anna was lying on the operating table as her surgeon came in, gowned, gloved and masked, his hands held carefully in front of him so as not to come into contact with anything that wasn't sterile. She couldn't see that Lachlan was smiling at her as he spoke but he hoped she might be able to hear it in his voice.

Anna's husband Clint was holding her hand. The anaesthetist was at her head, monitoring her spinal anaesthetic and the two IV lines that had been placed, one for fluids and the other for administering insulin and glucose to keep Anna's blood sugar stable. A scrub nurse was arranging instruments on the sterile surface of a trolley and others were pinning up the drapes to screen off the surgical field from the parents. Anna's midwife was also close.

'All set, Pippa?'

'Yes.'

Pippa met his gaze steadily. He couldn't tell if she was smiling because of her mask, but he *could* tell that she wasn't angry with him any longer. She was over trying to avoid him. There was something else in that split second of eye contact, but this was no time to wonder what effect sharing his story with her last night might have had.

Oddly, it hadn't thrown him into as dark a place as he'd expected. He could almost feel confident that he wasn't going to lose any newfound peace with his past—or his future? He might keep it very well hidden, but a part of him had always been prepared for the worst. If his test results were positive, he could still hope for the best for his baby and support Pippa in raising the child for as long as he possibly could. If his results were negative...

No. He wasn't going to let his mind go there, even for a nanosecond. Not just because he was about to focus completely on the surgery ahead of him but because he knew the fishhook that could be hidden in hope. Buried so deeply in your heart that when that hope was ripped away, it took far too much of your heart with it.

Pippa was all set. She had finished her preparations for this emergency C-section. All she needed to do now was to pick up the sterile towel and be ready to take the baby as soon as it was born. She was pleased to have her presence acknowledged and more than relieved to meet Lachlan's gaze. She hadn't seen him since he'd brought dinner to her cottage last night to share his harrowing story, and she'd had an almost sleepless night, not just feeling broken-hearted for him but worrying that he had far more reason than she'd ever had to prefer that they didn't work together.

There was no sign of him resenting her presence in Theatre, however. If anything, the way he had just acknowledged her felt as if there was a new connection between them. That anything private they knew about each other was exactly that. Private. It didn't have any bearing on them working together but it had inevitably deepened the level of trust between them.

Lachlan nodded at his team. 'Anna came in with the first signs of going into labour this afternoon and an ultrasound has revealed that, due to her high level of amniotic fluid, her baby has managed to get into a transverse lie, which is why it turns out today is going to be his birthday.' He held out his hand. 'Scalpel, please, Suzie.'

Pippa was aware of the concern regarding the effect of stress and the emergency surgery on Anna's blood sugar levels as well. Both she and the baby would be monitored very closely in the next twenty-four hours, and the sooner this surgery was safely over the better.

The first incision had been made through the skin and Lachlan was moving swiftly but surely as he navigated through muscle, fascia and the peritoneum to open the uterus. Pippa saw his hand going in and expected to see the baby emerging seconds later. Instead, she saw a small arm appear and then the frown lines on Lachlan's forehead deepened. He pushed the arm back inside and his whole hand disappeared into the incision. It seemed that the baby had managed to wedge itself into a difficult position.

'You're doing very well, Anna.' Lachlan's voice gave no hint of the effort he was putting into trying to extract this baby against a ticking clock. 'You're going to feel me doing a bit of pushing and pulling but it shouldn't be hurting.'

Pippa wasn't the only person to be glancing up at the clock. The length of time and how difficult it was to extract a baby could be a significant factor in a birth injury or worse, a fatality.

Lachlan was twisting his own body as he reached even further inside the abdomen.

'I'm just trying to find a foot,' he said. 'That's the only way to be sure I've followed the leg and not an arm. Ah…there it is.'

His hand appeared, two tiny ankles locked

between his gloved fingers. He was applying gentle traction and rotating the baby at the same time as he brought the legs out first and then the body of the baby boy. He lifted it up as the cord was clamped and cut and Pippa almost gasped.

The baby hung in his hands like a ragdoll, the head and limbs dangling, completely limp. Pippa took the infant into the towel she was holding and took it straight to the resuscitation unit.

'Page the Paeds team,' she heard Lachlan say behind her. 'They're on standby.'

The specialist neonatal team was in the theatre within what felt like only seconds. Pippa was still drying and trying to stimulate the baby. Someone ripped open a mask and another doctor had a stethoscope disc in place on the chest.

'Heart rate's just on a hundred,' they said.

The neonatal consultant was positioning the baby's head and clearing the airway with suction from a bulb syringe.

'Still not breathing,' she said.

The mask fitted over the nose and mouth completely. The ribs on the small chest were visible as it rose and fell with each rapid puff that was delivered.

The stethoscope was back in place as the seconds ticked past into a minute. Pippa was aware of more frequent glances coming in their direction from where the surgeon and his team were working to deliver the placenta and then close Anna's abdomen.

The first sound the baby made was like a bird chirping. And then it was a gargle. Finally, they could all hear the unmistakable sound of a newborn announcing his presence in the world and Pippa had never felt quite this relieved. She wrapped the baby up when the paediatric team were satisfied he was stable and she put a little woollen hat on his head to help keep him warm. Finally, she could take this precious bundle back to the operating table and show him to his parents. She held the baby close to Anna's face.

'He's gorgeous,' she told them. 'And he's absolutely fine. He was just a bit shocked at the way he had to come out.'

Pippa had been shocked, too.

And it hadn't been simply on a professional level. She had felt a connection to the baby in her own womb in that moment she'd seen the frightening limpness of the baby in Lachlan's hands.

She'd known, without giving it any conscious thought, in the split second before she took Anna's baby into her hands that she was going to fight for her own baby, no matter what battles might lie ahead. She was going to love it with all her heart and be the best mother she could be. For ever, hopefully. But certainly for as long as she possibly could, if fate had other plans in store for her or her child.

She was going to take a leaf out of Lachlan's book and live as if their baby was free of the disease. She would deal with whatever happened, if it happened, but until then she didn't want to know.

She did, however—at some point—need to let Lachlan know.

When Pippa told Lachlan a few days later that she needed to talk to him, he suggested a walk. Tomorrow, when they both had a day off. Well away from the hospital.

He drove them to Richmond Park and took a path that was still familiar, even after so many years.

'I learned to ride a bike here,' he told her. 'And I helped Liam learn to ride his. And that little forest of oak trees over there? That was our favourite spot for family picnics.'

It was where they stopped, grateful for a shady break from a surprisingly warm autumn afternoon.

'It looks like someone mowed the grass for us,' Pippa said as she sat down.

'More likely, it's been eaten down by the deer. We'll need to keep an eye out for them at this time of year. It's rutting season and the bucks can be more aggressive.'

'Is it safe to be here?'

'We'll hear them. Or see them. We can move away and keep our distance.' Lachlan smiled at her. 'I'll keep you safe, I promise. Although I'm not so sure about the weather. There are some rather black looking clouds not that far away.'

Pippa shrugged. 'What's the worst that could happen? We're not going to melt if we get a bit wet.'

'True.' Lachlan sat down beside her and tipped his head back to enjoy what was left of the sunshine streaming through leaves that were beginning to take on their autumn colours. 'What was it you wanted to talk to me about?'

'Um…the test.'

'I don't have the result yet. The DNA that gets extracted from the blood samples has to be sent to a specialised laboratory for analysis. It can take four to six weeks.'

Pippa nodded. 'Yes, you told me. But it's not your test I wanted to talk to you about. It's the baby's.'

'That will only need to be done if my result is positive.'

But Pippa shook her head. 'I don't want to have it done,' she said quietly. 'Even if your result *is* positive.'

Lachlan felt a chill run down his spine. He could feel his muscles tightening. Was it anger? That, again, she wasn't giving him a choice? Or was it fear—for his own diagnosis and then for that of his child?

His words were even quieter than Pippa's had been. 'Why not?'

'Because I don't want to know. I want to live in hope. Like you've been able to do…' Pippa was biting her bottom lip. 'Until I came along and made that impossible for you.'

Lachlan was still grappling with his emotional reaction to what she'd said.

'And there's another reason.'

'Which is?'

'There's a risk with having amniocentesis done. For miscarriage.'

'A very small risk. Less than one percent.'

'It's not a small risk for me.' Pippa wasn't looking at Lachlan now. She was letting her fingers drift through the blades of grass beside her. 'I've had miscarriages before,' she told him. 'Too many.'

Lachlan blinked. '*How* many?'

'Five…'

He swallowed. Hard. How could he have not had any idea of the kind of challenges Pippa had faced in her life?

How did she manage to find so much joy in delivering and being with other people's babies?

Why had he made a stupid joke about her husband leaving her for her obstetrician when the guy had just been rubbing salt in what had to be a gaping wound? Had the end of the marriage coincided with yet another unhappy end to a pregnancy?

It broke his heart to think that Pippa might have had to cope with that on her own.

'I had *no* idea,' he said slowly. 'I'm so sorry… I can't begin to imagine how hard that's been for you.'

Pippa's nod only acknowledged his sympathy. Her face was showing no expression. 'I never got past eleven weeks,' she said. 'And they never found a reason for it. I didn't have any abnormalities with my uterus. I didn't have any hormonal issues and there weren't any genetic problems. I'd never smoked and I gave up alcohol and coffee. I'm just one of the fifty percent or so of women who have recurrent miscarriages and never get to find out why.'

Lachlan let his breath out in a long, slow sigh. 'So that's why you waited so long to tell me that you were pregnant? Because you thought you wouldn't actually need to?'

Another nod.

'And then I got to twelve weeks, but I couldn't

believe that it was real. That was why I was doing that ultrasound on myself—the one you walked in on.' Pippa finally looked up. 'This is kind of a miracle to me,' she said. 'I tried for so long, again and again, despite the heartbreak, because it meant everything to me to have a baby. This wasn't supposed to happen. What are the odds of two forms of contraception failing at the same time? But it did happen and…it feels like it was meant to be.'

The odds were almost zero, Lachlan had to admit.

'I know I might have a terrible price to pay for being able to have this baby and love it with every bit of my heart.' Pippa had to pause and clear her throat. 'But I'm prepared to pay that price because…' He could hear a hitch in her voice now that suggested tears were even closer. 'Because that's what life is really all about, isn't it? Loving people? Taking that risk?'

A sudden gust of wind was a warning that the temperature was dropping fast as the sun went behind clouds. But was that the only reason why Lachlan felt a chill?

Hadn't he thought something along the same lines not that long ago? When he'd come to the point where he could embrace memories of his brother instead of avoiding them? When he'd realised that he wouldn't want to have missed that part of his life? Given the choice in hindsight, he had decided that the price was worth paying, so how could he blame Pippa for making that choice in advance?

But had he really missed what was *most* important about life? What about being the best person you could be? Or being the best doctor you could be and helping as many people as you could?

Pippa filled the silence. 'I know you don't feel like that and I understand why and…and I'm sad for you, but if I can keep this miracle going and carry this baby long enough, I'm going to love him or her enough for both of us.'

Lachlan still couldn't find any words. He was caught on the fact that she was feeling sorry for him. For what he was missing out on.

'I don't know what's going to happen,' Pippa said, her tone suggesting that she had said almost everything she wanted to. 'But… I can't throw hope away. For this pregnancy or for the future of my baby. I don't want the joy to be stolen from everything that happens in the next who knows how many years and… I know you can understand that because it's what you've chosen for yourself. And you can still do that. You don't have to tell me the results. You don't even have to find out yourself, if you can still be okay with that?'

Could he?

'I don't know,' he admitted. 'I'll have to think about that. It's different now.'

'Because of the baby?'

He nodded. 'It was absolutely better not to know for myself. But for a baby? Watching them grow up? Waiting for every milestone like that first smile and starting to walk and going to school or learning to ride a bike? Maybe I need to know, because otherwise the black cloud on the horizon that's always been there for myself will be so much bigger. And blacker. Close enough to block the sun, maybe—like those real clouds are doing at the moment.'

As if to join the conversation, those real clouds chose that moment to part and unleash more than a mere shower. Huge, fat raindrops began to fall, heavy enough for the leaves of the oak tree to offer little protection.

'Shall we wait it out or make a run for it?'

Pippa was already scrambling to her feet. 'We'll get far too cold if we try and wait it out.'

They got far too cold, anyway. And far too wet. Lachlan cranked the heater up when they got back to his car and headed straight for Pippa's cottage so that she could get dry and warm. She was shivering uncontrollably now despite the efficient heating of the car and the last thing he wanted was for her to end up getting sick. She had more than enough to deal with right now.

He got out of his car to make sure she got inside fast as well, because her hands were cold enough to be fumbling with her keys.

'Are you going to be okay?'

'I'm fine.'

But she didn't look fine. If she couldn't manage her key, how was she going to get her sodden clothes off and into a hot shower fast enough?

'I'm not convinced,' he said. 'And it was my idea to go on that walk. I'm coming in to make sure you *are* okay.'

He knew where the bathroom was. He knew how to turn on this shower because he'd done it before. On their first date.

On the night that Pippa had become pregnant.

Oh, God…she was fumbling with the metal fastener on her jeans now, her fingers shaking.

Lachlan could feel how slippery the slope he was stepping onto was, but he couldn't stop himself. He covered Pippa's hands with his own.

'Here…' The word came out as a kind of growl. 'Let me…'

He peeled the wet denim off her legs. And then she held her arms up like a child so he could lift the wet shirt over her head. The small bathroom was filling with steam as she stood there in her bra and knickers and Lachlan knew this was when he should step out, but he couldn't move. His gaze ran down Pippa's body. There was no hint of a pregnancy bump yet but she looked different, somehow.

Even more gorgeous than she had on that first date. Or the second...

She was looking up at him, water dripping from her hair to trickle down her face. Her lips were parted and her eyes were so dark—her pupils dilated with...desire, that was what he could see.

What he could feel in every cell in his own body.

An intense desire that felt like flames licking his skin and made him shiver.

'You're cold, too,' Pippa whispered. 'You can share my shower.'

Pippa had never had sex in a shower before.

She'd never had sex knowing that she was pregnant, either.

Or when she was cold enough for the hot water to feel as if it was burning her skin, and Lachlan's hands were cold enough to be creating an oddly similar kind of burn. Together, the sensations were unbelievable. Like the rain of hot water on her face as it was tilted up to meet Lachlan's lips and what felt like a ripple effect when the heat of his tongue met hers. How wet their bodies were and the slide of hands that were slippery with shower gel was another dimension that was off any charts that might record physical arousal, or satisfaction.

It was, without doubt, *the* most astonishing sex she'd ever had.

Scorchingly hot. Astonishingly intense. And over far too soon.

It seemed like Lachlan was thinking the same thing because when they'd almost exhausted her supply of hot water, he wrapped them both in towels and then carried her to her bed to do it all over again.

This was where it had all started.

And this had to be where it all ended, didn't it?

There was something very poignant about the smile that Lachlan gave her after a slow, exquisitely tender kiss a long time later.

'I guess this counts as date number three,' he murmured.

Pippa's huff of laughter could almost have been a tiny sob.

'I guess it does.'

CHAPTER THIRTEEN

THE LATER IT GOT, the more tempting it became to let his mind wander.

Lachlan Smythe was in his office, trying to get a presentation on high-risk pregnancies ready as a guest speaker for an upcoming midwifery conference.

He had a well-drawn, colourful illustration of the anatomy of the uterus on his computer screen and he was adding arrows and text that would appear with a click of a mouse, to make it a slide for the presentation. He was recording prompts on another document to make sure he didn't leave out any of the key information he wanted to impart.

'Here we have the three layers of the uterus,' he said aloud, as he typed into the second document. 'The endometrium on the inside, the myometrium in the middle and the perimetrium on the outside. The endometrium is where the placenta is implanted, and what I'm going to talk about today is where this implantation can go wrong and result in placenta accreta, increta and percreta.'

He needed to start a new slide to describe the different degrees that a placenta could grow past a normal implantation, but it was a word he'd just said that continued to hang in the air, like the aftermath of a bell tolling.

Okay…his focus was gone but the word was still there.

…*wrong*…

Wrong, wrong, wrong.

Had he been following an ill-advised track in his personal life, for the whole of his adult life? Pippa seemed to think so and it had prompted him, over the last couple of days, to think more about his philosophy on living than he had since he'd been an angsty teenager, grappling with the meaning of life as he'd navigated the grief of losing his brother and then having to watch his father pulled slowly away by the appalling grip of Huntington's Disease.

Pippa hadn't experienced that, so it was all very well for her to tell him that the most important thing in life was having people to love and that it was sad that he felt he had to keep others at a safe emotional distance, but she had no idea what she could actually be facing in the future, did she? No idea at all.

Lachlan rubbed at his forehead with his fingers.

'The recognised risk factors for developing accreta lie with scarring of the endometrium from previous Caesarean sections or surgery for fibroids,' he said, redirecting his focus yet again. 'Or due to a placenta praevia, where the placenta has attached itself to the lower segment of the uterus where the walls are thinner.'

He was typing bullet points onto the slide as he spoke, trying to ignore an insistent unrelated thought that was doing its best to disrupt the flow.

A voice that was asking him how on earth he had come to the conclusion that Pippa had no idea at all about grief?

She'd lost five babies.

Five.

He knew better than to dismiss the degree of emotional fallout because she'd never got past her first trimester. She'd been dreaming of having a baby and she'd had to grieve the loss of both the baby and the future as a mother that she wanted so desperately every time every one of those pregnancies had failed.

She'd been brave enough to try again, though, hadn't she?

Again and again.

Until, to add insult to injury, she'd found her husband was cheating on her—with, presumably, the person who was treating her recurrent miscarriages—and she'd lost her marriage as well.

Which was why she'd subscribed to that 'three date' rule, of course. And why he'd felt so safe to play the game with her. She had been just as reluctant as he was to engage with someone on an intimate level.

But she was prepared to risk far more than the fallout of a relationship that hadn't worked. The future she was actually hoping she could face was a much bigger deal.

There was a baby involved.

A baby that might—or might not—one day have to face the decisions that were playing havoc with Lachlan's concentration right now. Because thinking about Pippa raised an even bigger temptation.

That he could take up her suggestion to cancel the testing process and keep living the way he always had.

With hope...

It would be a perfectly acceptable thing to do as far as the genetic clinic staff were concerned. You were allowed to pull out of the process at any point.

But if Lachlan did that he would be stealing the potential joy that would be there for Pippa if the result showed that he didn't have Huntington's himself and couldn't have passed it on to a baby. Pippa would never have to live with the cloud he'd been under for as long as he could remember and his own cloud would evaporate. Just like that. Poof!

A whole new world could open up for him.

One where he could allow himself to fall in love. To *be* loved. To have a whole family of his own, which was something he'd never allowed himself to dream of.

And, if that was the case, it would be Pippa that he would choose to share his life with. That was a given.

But it was a flip of a coin. And the other side from that joy was the grim confirmation of a slow death sentence that would also open up a whole new world he would have to step into.

The circle of his thoughts always came back to the same question. Was it really better to live with hope for as long as possible? Or, as Pippa had suggested, was he only living half a life and missing the most important part?

With a sigh, Lachlan hit save on the work he'd started and then shut down his laptop. He'd go into the diagnosis and management of placental tissue that could grow far enough to escape the uterus and invade the bladder later—maybe when he got home. Part of this presentation would be covering the massive blood loss that could happen with attempting the removal of a placenta accreta and it was even more likely to make him think about Pippa and that dramatic night they'd first met if he was still here in his office.

And thinking about Pippa would only lead his tired brain back onto the same path that just kept going round in the same loop. It wasn't as if he actually had a choice. Because this wasn't just about him any longer. Pippa might not want to know what the future held but, to Lachlan, it felt like part of his responsibility as a father. How could you protect someone to the best of your ability if you didn't know what you might be up against?

Lachlan could hear the raised voices as soon as he left his office and he felt the hairs on the back of his neck rise. Violence against hospital staff was increasing everywhere and the labour ward had its fair share of abusive and uncooperative patients and relatives. He'd been told they had a great security team at Queen Mary's, but nobody could be everywhere at once and trouble in the emergency department could mean that these well-trained guards were unavailable in other areas of the hospital.

He lengthened his stride as he heard the aggressive note in a male voice. It sounded as if it was coming from the reception desk that was just inside the entrance to the ward. Rita would be at that desk and the thought of their motherly and warm-hearted receptionist being subjected to abuse like this was totally unacceptable.

'Don't tell me you don't have the keys. I *know* you've got them—you're just being a bitch...'

A crashing sound came just as Lachlan turned into the reception area. Rita was looking terrified. The computer screen that was normally in front of her had been pulled across the desk, ripped free of its cables and was lying on the floor.

'My girlfriend *needs* drugs.' A tall, very skinny man in ripped jeans and a hoodie started swearing at Rita. 'She's having a *baby*. Everybody gets drugs when they're having babies. The stupid nurse isn't getting them fast enough so, guess what? Turns out it's your job...'

Rita jumped back from the desk as he reached across the desk to grab her. She saw Lachlan coming and cried out.

The man's head swung around and Lachlan saw the spiderweb tattoos across his face and the piercings in his eyebrows and nose. There were two large spikes on either side of his mouth, below his bottom lip.

'Who the hell are *you*?'

Lachlan saw Rita picking up a phone. He

knew she would be calling for help. He just needed to buy some time.

'I'm a doctor. What's the problem here?'

'A *doctor*, huh…?'

The man was suddenly very still, his eyes narrowed. It felt as if a bomb was about to be detonated. Without moving his own head, Lachlan scanned the area around them. There was no sign of any of the night shift staff. No sign of anyone else. What he could see, against the wall beside him, was an abandoned wheelchair.

The trigger came when shouting could be heard coming from Room Three. As the man launched himself in Lachlan's direction, he grabbed the handles of the chair to put in front of him as a barrier. When he saw the man pulling out a knife, he shoved the wheelchair forward and the metal footplates smacked into his legs. The man shrieked in pain but stepped back, looking over his shoulder as if he expected an attack from behind as well. He had to be able to hear Rita shouting into the phone as clearly as Lachlan could. He would be able to see the face on the other side of the doors that needed swipe cards or for Rita to deactivate the lock from the desk. Sally must have been coming back from a break and she was staring through the glass panels of the doors, horrified.

The man with the knife in his hand could see

that there were people on three sides of him. With another stream of profanity, he took off in the only direction that was clear. He wrenched the first door he came to so hard Lachlan could hear wood splintering as he slammed it shut behind him.

Lachlan ran towards Rita. 'Are you okay?'

Her nod was jerky.

'Have you called Security?'

She nodded again. 'They're on their way.'

Another glance at the door showed that Sally had turned her head. Was she watching the arrival of the security guards?

'Is his girlfriend in Room Three?' That was the best place for them both to be.

'Yes…' But Rita's voice was a frightened whisper. 'So's Pippa…'

The knot that suddenly formed in Lachlan's gut was tight enough to cause pain. Big enough to stop him being able to take a proper breath. He wasn't going to wait for anyone else to arrive.

He couldn't.

Pippa was in trouble and protecting her had just become the thing that mattered most in his life.

The only thing that mattered…?

They were drug seekers.

The woman, Kardi, *was* probably six months

pregnant but she wasn't in labour, despite her dramatic entrance to the labour ward a short time ago, clutching her belly and screaming in pain, with a man helping her to stay upright. Pippa was walking through the reception area, on her way back from the staff toilet, when Rita had opened the door to the panicked request of the new arrivals and she'd had no choice but to take them straight into a room to assess the situation. The screaming had to be upsetting everybody, including the woman Pippa was caring for in Room Two that she'd only intended to be away from for a minute or two.

'Can you get Sally or anyone else that's free to come and help, please, Rita?'

'Sally's on her break but I'll find someone.'

But nobody had arrived and Pippa knew she might be in trouble as soon as she was alone in Room Three with the couple.

'I'm Pippa, one of the midwives here. What's your name?'

'Kardi. With a K.'

She'd stopped screaming. The man with her was standing with his back to the door of the room.

'Let's get you into a gown and up on the bed so I can see what's happening. How far along in your pregnancy are you?'

'Dunno. 'Bout seven months.' She moved towards the bed but stopped to bend forward and groan loudly. 'It *really* hurts. Where's the gas?'

'You need more than gas, sweetheart,' her companion said. 'Morphine. That's what you need.'

'Yeah…that's what I need. Or methadone'll do. Haven't had enough today, you know?'

Pippa managed to sound much calmer than she was feeling. She opened a cupboard to find a gown. 'Put this on, Kardi. I'll get you comfortable and then I'll go and find a doctor. I can sign off on any drugs like that.' She put the gown down on the end of the bed. 'I can see you're in real pain,' she said. 'Let me go and call a doctor now.'

She turned towards the door, only to find that Kardi's partner was standing right in her way.

'You're not going anywhere,' the man said. 'Kardi, you come and watch the door. I'll go and get what we're here for. Give this nurse a kicking if she tries to go anywhere, right?'

'Yeah…go on. Hurry up.' Kardi turned back to Pippa. 'So…where's the gas, then?'

'Right here.' Pippa pointed to the other side of the bed. 'I'll set it up for you, shall I?'

She edged carefully around the end of the bed, knowing she could be attacked at any time. She didn't have to look over her shoulder to know that the door of the en-suite bathroom was open.

Pippa knew there was a lock on the door. Not that it was ever used, but it seemed that bathroom doors automatically came with a locking system. Kardi's attention was on the mouthpiece she was taking from its sterile packaging. Holding her breath, Pippa turned as if she was about to find the tubing to attach the mouthpiece to, but she dropped it on the bed instead, ran into the bathroom and shut the door behind her. She twisted the lock just as Kardi started banging on the door.

She heard another door banging only seconds later. And shouting, from the two people in the room—at each other, as they realised their plan was going wrong—and from outside the room. Male voices. Pippa could only hope they were from Security, but she was so terrified her mind was playing tricks on her and she could almost imagine that one of those voices was Lachlan's. Then it was drowned by the thumping of someone's body slamming the bathroom door.

'Open it!' The command was a scream.

Pippa had been leaning against the door from the inside, but feeling it move made her retreat until she had a solid wall behind her back. She slid down to sit in the small space between the toilet and the shower and squeezed her eyes shut.

She might die, she thought. If these violent drug seekers got to her first. She could hear

Lachlan's voice again then. From just the other day, when they were in the park and she'd been a bit nervous about the possibility of being amongst male deer in the rutting season.

I'll keep you safe, I promise…

If only…

But thinking about it was enough to comfort her. And thank goodness he wouldn't be here at this time of night.

Except he did stay late sometimes, didn't he? Pippa's mind was racing now, back in time. It had been in this room that he'd arrived like a knight in shining armour to rescue her from a situation that had been so scary.

Not as scary as this one, though…

Pippa put her hands over her ears. She couldn't bear the crashing sounds and shouting that was going on out there. She could still hear it, though it was getting steadily quieter, fading into the distance.

Until there was silence.

Pippa's heart skipped a beat as someone tried the door handle.

'Pippa?'

It was Lachlan. And she could hear the fear in his voice.

'Are you okay? Can you open the door? You're safe… I promise…'

CHAPTER FOURTEEN

THIS...

The moment he could take Pippa into his arms and hold her so tightly he couldn't tell where his body ended and hers started.

This *feeling...*

It was bigger than anything. Bigger than *everything*.

'Oh, my God, Pippa... I thought... I thought I might have lost you.'

He could feel her trembling in his arms. When Sally, with a security officer right behind her, came to the door of the bathroom, Lachlan gave his head a tiny shake and mouthed that it was okay.

He had this.

Sally looked from Lachlan to Pippa and back again. She turned and walked away, forcing the security officer behind her to move far enough away so that she could shut the door quietly. She had a rather misty smile on her face, as if she knew exactly how big this moment was for Lachlan.

And for Pippa?

Lachlan's lips were against Pippa's hair. 'I can't lose you,' he whispered. He pressed his lips to her hair. 'I love you.'

Pippa's words were muffled because she was still pressed so hard against his chest. 'I love you, too,' she said. 'I thought I was going to die and all I wanted was...*you*. And I could remember you telling me that you were going to keep me safe and... I just played that over and over in my mind and...' Her voice was choked with tears. 'I *did* feel safe...'

Lachlan knew his own voice was thick with the overwhelming emotion that had pushed its way through what now seemed like flimsy barriers protecting his heart.

'But I can't...' He hauled in a breath before saying the words he least wanted to say. 'I might *not* be able to keep you safe. Or give you a future.'

Pippa lifted her head. Her eyes looked huge in her pale, tear-streaked face but the look in them was melting something inside Lachlan.

His fear?

'You're giving me *this*,' she told him softly. 'This moment. And it's the biggest and best moment of my entire life. And even if I never had another moment like this, it would be worth it because I can remember it for ever and—' She pulled in a distinctly shaky sounding breath. 'If I ever have another moment where I think I'm not going to be alive much longer, *this* is what I'm going to remember. You telling me that you loved me and me saying it back and that—in that moment—life couldn't have been any more perfect.'

She was right, Lachlan realised with absolute certainty. Life *was* made up of moments and the best ones were…priceless. They became memories that could be treasured for as long as you lived. But the others…?

'Could you take that risk?' he asked quietly. 'That there might be a limit to moments like this?'

'I thought I was never going to have *this* one.' Pippa was smiling through her tears now. 'And I'm going to kiss you now and that's going to be another one.'

Lachlan started to dip his head. He wanted that kiss too. *So* much…

But Pippa pulled back in his arms, just enough to keep their eye contact.

'We'll make the most of every moment,' she said. 'For as long as we can. It's all anyone can do, isn't it? It's just that some people have more idea of what could be around the corner and…

and maybe that's not such a bad thing, because every moment like this will make us realise how lucky we are. And...' Her eyes widened, as though she'd just had an even better idea. 'If you really love someone, doesn't that mean that you don't leave them to face bad stuff alone?'

She loved him *that* much? That she wouldn't want him to be facing the bad stuff by himself?

He could see the answer to that in her eyes. He could feel it in his heart at the same time because...because he loved *her* that much. And she was right. He would never want her to face anything that could be distressing without him being close enough to comfort her.

Lachlan could taste the salt of tears on Pippa's lips but he didn't know if they were his tears or hers.

Not that it mattered. They had this moment and he could only hope that this kiss was making Pippa feel as cherished and...hopeful...as he was feeling.

When a polite knock on the door reminded him that there was rather a lot of witness statements and paperwork and finding replacement staff to cover the rest of this night shift that needed to be done in the wake of a major incident in the department he was the head of, he ignored it.

Just long enough to make this moment last for another heartbeat.

The next knock was louder.

'Are you guys okay in there?'

'We're good,' Lachlan called. 'We'll be out in just a second.'

He needed that second.

He smiled at Pippa. 'I think I need a date.'

'A *fourth* date?' Her eyebrows rose. 'You do know that's breaking the rules, don't you?'

His smile widened. 'Not a fourth date. I mean an actual date. On a calendar. The kind you can draw a circle around.'

'But is it a date for a date?'

'No…' Lachlan's smile wobbled, just a little. 'A date for our wedding. If you'll marry me, that is?'

Pippa caught her bottom lip between her teeth, but her arms tightened around Lachlan's neck and she was coming up on her tiptoes, clearly intent on kissing him again.

'I think that's actually in the rule book,' she murmured. 'The fourth date is for the proposal and the answer is always yes.'

That worked for Lachlan.

He was more than happy to ask the big question again. He'd have a perfect ring ready because Pippa could help him choose it. He'd go down on one knee and he'd know the things he really wanted to say so that he could tell Pippa the whole long list of every reason he loved her this much.

And how she had changed his life, because he was going to make the most of every special moment. He could look back and find comfort in moments from the past and he wouldn't look too far ahead because they weren't there yet and why would you spoil something as perfect as what was happening right now?

Another blink of time stolen from the world outside.

Another kiss.

The envelope had been there for weeks now.

On the desk at home, hidden under a pile of medical journals that were still waiting to be read because life had been so very busy.

Pippa had moved into Lachlan's new house and they'd had a wedding to prepare for that had turned out to be the best day ever. Even the weather had cooperated enough to allow them to go and have their wedding photographs taken in Richmond Park, and the one he would treasure for ever was under the now bare branches of that huge oak tree, with Pippa in her gorgeous white dress on a carpet of autumn leaves, some of them red enough to be an echo of her hair that was hanging in ringlets as Lachlan was tipping her back to kiss his bride yet again.

He'd forgotten completely about the envelope that day. He hadn't thought about it during the week they'd been on honeymoon on a gorgeous Greek island, either.

But they were home again and settling into their new life together and…he was almost ready. He hadn't been ready when the results of his test had become available. He'd been offered another counselling session at the Genetics Centre to discuss the results but he'd declined. What he did request was to have the results sent to him so that he could open the envelope in his own time.

On his own.

Because when he'd had the phone call to say that they had arrived, he'd come to what felt like a compromise he could live with in an ethical dilemma that was so difficult to resolve.

At some point soon, Lachlan needed to know so that he could prepare for the future in a way that meant he could protect the people he loved the most.

Pippa.

And their daughter. He'd felt the baby move last night for the first time, his hand resting gently on Pippa's now noticeably rounded belly.

They'd agreed to avoid even the slight risk

to the pregnancy that the amniocentesis represented. They would live in hope for this baby.
Even if Lachlan was carrying the gene, there
was still a fifty percent chance that their baby
would not be. The odds of a paediatric form of
the disease were low enough to be acceptable
and who knew what advances in medicine could
happen in the decades to come? Lachlan couldn't
steal the hope that was shining in Pippa's face
as she put her hand over his to feel the kick of
tiny feet, or maybe it was the prod of an elbow.
A nudge to remind them to make the most of
another one of those moments.

No. He wasn't going to steal that hope.

But he was going to find out the result. Because he needed to know. And if he was clear,
he could offer Pippa more than simply hope.

He could give her the gift of making the sun
shine brightly enough to blitz those black clouds
and give them both the clear skies that most
other people got to live with.

If he wasn't clear, he wasn't going to tell
Pippa.

That would make the hope she was living with
his gift instead. He could keep the result hidden for as long as possible because he loved her
that much.

When he was sure Pippa was asleep, Lachlan
slipped quietly out of bed and put his bathrobe

on. He went to his study and turned on the desk lamp. He pulled the envelope out from under the journals and held it in his hands.

For a long, long moment, he stared at it. Taking in a very deep breath.

Steadying himself.

The soft voice at the door made the breath leave his lungs in a rush.

'Is that what I think it is?' Pippa asked.

'Yes.'

'You were going to open it without me?'

Lachlan's heart broke at what he could see in her eyes.

'I didn't want you to know,' he said quietly. 'If it was bad news.'

'That's not fair...' Pippa came closer. 'If you get to protect me and I can't do the same for you.' She held out her hand. 'I love you, Lachlan,' she said steadily. 'And my life is in that envelope as much as yours is.' Her voice dropped to a whisper. 'Let me open it?'

Lachlan couldn't say anything past the lump in his throat. Silently, he handed the envelope to Pippa.

She opened it and withdrew a single sheet of paper.

And then she stared at it.

Frowning.

Lachlan felt the world stop turning. 'It's bad news, isn't it?'

'I don't know,' Pippa said. 'I don't understand. What are CAG repeats?'

'It's a DNA code for the chemicals that the Huntington's gene contains. Most people have a level that's low enough that they're not at risk for the disease. Some are a bit higher, which means they're not likely to get the disease themselves but they could still pass it on to their children. If they're really high they already have it and, the higher the level, the younger it can start.'

'Okay. So that range is the twenty-seven to thirty-six repeats in the brackets here.'

'Yes.'

'So…' Pippa looked up, her eyes filling with tears as she held the piece of paper out to Lachlan. 'Twelve is good, yes…?'

Dazed, Lachlan looked at the result.

There it was, in black and white.

He was clear. He was not going to get the disease and there was no way their baby could be affected.

The clouds were breaking apart and vanishing but they were leaving a few drops of rain behind.

Or were they tears?

Of joy?

That was certainly what it felt like as Lachlan

wrapped Pippa in his arms, the paper slipping through his fingers to drift to the floor.

This was another one of those moments.

And it felt like the biggest one yet.

EPILOGUE

Four months later...

'LACHLAN? ARE YOU AWAKE?'

'I am now, darling.' Lachlan snapped on a bedside light and propped himself up on one elbow. 'Are you okay?'

'Um… I got up to go to the loo but then this happened…'

Pippa was standing in the door of the master bedroom's en-suite bathroom. She was wearing a soft tee shirt that was pushed up so far by her belly that the elastic waistband of the silky boxer shorts she was wearing as well was visible. Pale pink shorts that Lachlan could see had a dark stain on them that was growing rapidly bigger. He dropped his gaze and…yes…there was a puddle on the floor where Pippa was standing.

'Your waters have broken.'

'You think?' Pippa grinned. 'Thank goodness I married an obstetrician.'

Lachlan was out of bed. He pulled a jumper

on and then reached for his jeans. 'We'd better get going. Where's your bag? How far apart are your contractions?'

'Haven't had one yet. Oh…wait.' Pippa was biting her lip as Lachlan pulled up his jeans. She let out a groan as she released her breath. 'Yep… that's a contraction, all right.'

'Thank goodness I married a midwife.' But Lachlan wasn't smiling. He looked, Pippa decided, rather adorably scared stiff.

She had to cling onto the door frame then, to ride out the rest of an unexpectedly strong contraction. Had she somehow slept through hours of the early stages of her labour?

'What do you want to wear?' Lachlan asked. 'To go to the hospital?' He turned back to pick up his phone. 'I'd better let them know we're on our way.'

'Not yet.' Pippa blew out a breath as the pain finally began to subside. 'The first thing Rita's going to ask is how far apart my contractions are. *Oh*…'

'What? What is it? What's wrong?' Lachlan was right beside her and Pippa grabbed hold of his arm instead of the door frame.

'Another…contraction…' she gasped. '*Oh-h*…'

The pain was fierce. Back-to-back with the last contraction. It was then that Pippa realised they weren't going to make it to the birthing suite at Queen Mary's. Despite being a partnership of an obstetrician and a midwife, they'd never even considered a home birth. Possibly because they both wanted to be in the safest possible place for the arrival of what felt like the most precious baby in the world.

Pippa felt her knees giving way beneath her. Lachlan took her weight until she was safely on the floor, on her hands and knees.

'I need to check your dilation,' he said. 'Don't push, okay…?'

'I don't think I need to,' Pippa groaned. 'Get my shorts off. I can feel the baby's head… I *need* to push…'

'No…wait.' Lachlan's voice was a command. Authoritative. Calm.

Pippa could feel her clothing being removed. She could feel his hands on her body. She could feel pressure. Lachlan was pushing back on the baby's head. Trying to slow the delivery. She could feel another contraction beginning to build and she put all her focus into not giving in to the urge to push, opening her mouth and taking short, rapid breaths. How many times had she coached women to pant like this to try and slow labour down to prevent tearing or provide the chance to check that an umbilical cord wasn't wrapped around a baby's neck?

'You're doing great, hon,' Lachlan said. 'Oh, man…she's not to going wait, is she? Here we go…'

Pippa gave in to the push, knowing that the safest pair of hands imaginable were waiting to catch her baby. When had Lachlan had time to grab one of the towels from the bathroom? And how did he manage to turn her so that she was now sitting on the floor, ready to take her baby into her arms and hold her against her breasts? It was all a bit of a blur for a while then. She was shivering almost as much as she had been the day that they'd got caught in the rain.

No hot shower for her this time. Lachlan ripped the duvet off the bed and wrapped that around her. He'd called an ambulance.

'They've got an ETA of about five minutes,' he told Pippa.

'That's okay… We're fine…'

Their daughter wasn't crying, but she was breathing well and moving her arms and legs. She lay in her mother's arms and her eyes were wide open. She was simply lying on Pippa's skin and looking up at both her parents.

'Aren't you gorgeous?' Lachlan whispered. 'As gorgeous as your mum.'

Pippa looked up for the first time since she'd been given her baby to hold. She looked straight into the eyes of her baby's father as she leaned back into the circle of his arms.

'I love you,' she said softly.

'I love *you*.' Lachlan pressed a soft kiss onto Pippa's head. 'I can hear the ambulance arriving. I'll have to run downstairs and let them in.'

But he didn't move for a moment. And Pippa didn't want him to.

The realisation that they had just become a family was sinking in. They both looked down at their daughter. They had chosen her name long ago.

'Welcome to the world, Hope,' Pippa whispered. 'We love you, too.'

* * * * *

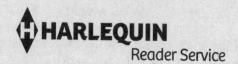
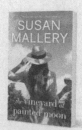
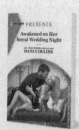
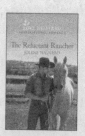
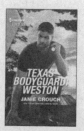